Founded in 1972, the Institute for Research on Public policy is an independent, national, nonprofit organization. Its mission is to improve public policy in Canada by promoting and contributing to a policy process that is more broadly based, informed and effective.

In pursuit of this mission, the IRPP

- identifies significant public-policy questions that will confront Canada in the longer term future, and undertakes independent research into these questions;
- promotes wide dissemination of key results from its own and other research activities;
- encourages non-partisan discussion and criticism of public policy issues by eliciting broad participation from all sectors and regions of Canadian society and linking research with processes of social learning and policy formation.

The IRPP's independence is assured by an endowment fund, to which federal and provincial governments and the private sector have contributed.

Créé en 1972, l'Institut de recherche en politiques publiques est un organisme national et indépendant à but non lucratif.

L'IRPP a pour mission de favoriser le développement de la pensée politique au Canada par son appui et son apport à un processus élargi, plus éclairé et plus efficace d'élaboration et d'expression des politiques publiques.

Dans le cadre de cette mission, l'IRPP a pour mandat :

- d'identifier les questions politiques auxquelles le Canada sera confronté dans l'avenir et d'entreprendre des recherches indépendantes à leur sujet;
- de favoriser une large diffusion des résultats les plus importants de ses propres recherches et de celles des autres sur ces questions;
- de promouvoir une analyse et une discussion objectives des questions politiques de manière à faire participer activement au débat public tous les secteurs de la société canadienne et toutes les régions du pays, et à rattacher la recherche à l'évolution sociale et à l'élaboration de politiques.

L'indépendance de l'IRPP est assurée par les revenus d'un fonds de dotation auquel ont souscrit les gouvernements fédéral et provinciaux, ainsi que le secteur privé.

The Brookings Institution is a private nonprofit organization devoted to research, education and publication on important issues of domestic and foreign policy. Its principal purpose is to bring knowledge to bear on current and emerging policy problems. The Institution was founded on December 8, 1927, to merge the activities of the Institute for Government Research, founded in 1916, the Institute of Economics, founded in 1922 and the Robert Brookings Graduate School of Economics, founded in 1924.

The Institution maintains a position of neutrality on issues of public policy. Interpretations or conclusions in Brookings publications should be understood to be solely those of the authors.

La « Brookings Institution » est un organisme privé, sans but lucratif. Sur les grandes questions de politique nationale ou étrangère, elle s'emploie à la recherche et à l'enseignement, ainsi qu'à la publication d'études. Son principal rôle est de favoriser la connaissance des problèmes actuels et de ceux qui se dessinent. Créée le 8 décembre 1927, la « Brookings Institution » fusionnait les activités de trois organismes préexistants : l'« Institute for Government Research » fondé en 1916, l'« Institute of Economics » fondé en 1922, et la « Robert Brookings Graduate School of Economics » fondée en 1924.

Sur toutes les questions de politiques publiques, la « Brookings Institution » conserve une stricte neutralité. Les auteurs des textes qu'elle publie assument l'entière responsabilité de leurs interprétations ou de leurs conclusions.

HEALTH CARE REFORM

THROUGH INTERNAL MARKETS:

EXPERIENCE AND PROPOSALS

———

Printed in Canada
Bibliothèque nationale du Québec - Dépôt légal 1995

CANADIAN CATALOGUING IN PUBLICATION DATA

Main entry under title:

Health care reform through internal markets :
experience and proposals

Most papers were presented at a conference,
Health Care Cost Control: Internal Market Mechanisms,
held in Montreal in May 1994.
Co-published by the Brookings Institution.
Includes preliminaries in English and French.
Includes bibliographical references.
ISBN 0-88645-162-0 (IRPP)
ISBN 0-8157-9365-0 (Brookings Institution)

1. Medical care—Cost control—Congresses.
2. Health care reform—Congresses. I. Jérôme-Forget, Monique II. White, Joseph
III. Wiener, Joshua M. IV. Institute for Research on Public Policy. V. Brookings Institution.

RA410.A2H43 1995   338.4'33621   C95-900061-5

Marye Ménard-Bos
Director of Publications, IRPP

—————————

Copy Editing: Jane Broderick

Design and Production: Schumacher Design
Cover Illustration: Geneviève Côté

Published by
The Institute for Research on Public Policy (IRPP)
1470 Peel Street, Suite 200
Montreal, Quebec H3A 1T1
and
The Brookings Institution
1775 Massachusetts Avenue, N.W.
Washington, D.C. 20036-2188

Distributed by
Renouf Publishing Co. Ltd.
1294 Algoma Road
Ottawa, Ontario K1B 3W8
Tel. 613-741-4333
Fax 613-741-5439

Contents

3

ACKNOWLEDGEMENTS

The conference and this publication could not have proceeded without the tireless efforts of many individuals at the Institute for Research on Public Policy (IRPP) and the Brookings Institution.

At IRPP, Marye Ménard-Bos, Director of Administration, and Chantal Létourneau ensured that both the conference and the production of this volume proceeded smoothly. Paula Ghazi, Director of Finance, Louise Dubuc, and Annamaria Verdicchio also made important contributions. Thor Sigvaldason provided excellent research and editorial assistance.

Mathew Horsman and Carole Sullivan of IRPP's magazine, *Policy Options/Options politiques,* laid the groundwork for the conference by devoting their October 1993 issue to the theme of health care reform. Mathew also provided editorial advice regarding the paper written at IRPP.

Elisabeth Reynolds deserves special mention for assisting us in putting together the conference agenda and lining up experts from around the world to deliver papers. She then coordinated the initial stages of the publishing process. Adil Sayeed replaced Elisabeth when she embarked on a course of graduate studies.

At the Brookings Institution, Cindy Terrels, Carole Plowfield, Anthony J. Sheehan, and Colette Solpietro provided invaluable assistance.

Finally, Jane Broderick provided quality editing and Jenny Schumacher and Natalie Coté met their usual standards of excellence in designing the publication.

Monique Jérôme-Forget
Institute for Research on Public Policy
Montréal

Joseph White
Joshua Wiener
The Brookings Institution
Washington, DC

MONIQUE JÉRÔME-FORGET,

JOSEPH WHITE AND JOSHUA M. WIENER

INTRODUCTION

Access to quality health care is important to every individual. Health care systems constitute major portions of every advanced industrial economy. Therefore, health care policy is a major responsibility for the governments of all those nations.

We are currently in an era of international health care reform. In spite of the many differences among the world's various systems, reform proposals everywhere are influenced by two concerns: the total cost of care, as a burden on the economy or on private or public budgets; and whether systems are providing "value for money" and thus whether they can be managed more efficiently. In the United States these issues are then joined with a conflict that has been settled everywhere else — over how and even whether to guarantee access to health care for all citizens. In other countries access is an issue because of concerns about how pursuit of cost control and efficiency might affect access as well as other values, such as quality.

Many countries are pursuing reform through the creation of "internal markets." The theory of internal markets departs from traditional "market-oriented" approaches to health care cost control, such as charging the patient directly. Advocates of internal markets believe that competition among health care providers can be introduced in such a way

---

that it does not threaten equity of access. The internal markets described in this book are not explicitly intended to threaten pre-existing structures of redistributive financing or of overall cost control.

The internal market model takes many forms, as the following papers will show. One example involves the dismantling of existing health care bureaucracies; instead of all the hospitals in an area being part of a larger organization, they would be managed separately and would compete for business from the paying organization in a "purchaser-provider split." In another form, deriving inspiration from American Health Maintenance Organizations (HMOs), individuals would be entitled to choose among groups of providers that would contract to provide all or some portion of care.

In most countries, internal markets are promoted as a means of allowing a public system to deliver health care efficiently within an overall cost cap. The exception is the US, where a cousin of the internal market idea, "managed competition," has been advocated mainly by those who vehemently reject a cap; the Clinton Administration, however, called for "managed competition with a global budget."

In its more usual forms, which have been adopted to some extent in a number of countries examined in this book, internal markets are intended to efficiently allocate a resource total that has been decided by a political process. To the extent that internal markets can do more with less, restrained expenditure increases should be easier to justify politically. Proponents also suggest that internal markets will result in increased patient influence over the provision of health care services.

The internal market approach has hardly been greeted with unanimous approval, however. Sceptics caution that advocates promise more than they can deliver. Difficult technical problems such as "risk selection" may have to be solved before the efficiency benefits of internal markets can be fully and safely realized. Internal health care markets will inevitably require extensive government regulation. In some cases, internal market competition may restrict the freedom of patients to choose their own doctors and hospitals (as the HMO model in the US does).

The Institute for Research on Public Policy and the Brookings Institution hoped to further this debate by sponsoring a conference on internal health care markets. This volume presents papers delivered at that conference, which was held in Montreal in May 1994. (The paper by Howard Glennerster, who was not a participant, is included to provide an overview of the British reforms and to describe the principles under-lying the internal market system.)

THE EUROPEAN EXPERIENCE WITH INTERNAL MARKETS

Internal market reforms have been implemented in Sweden, Finland, the Netherlands and the United Kingdom. The first five chapters review the European experience with internal markets. These papers reveal a great deal about the logic of internal market systems and the forms that internal markets have taken, as well as the potential benefits and risks of this approach.

Howard Glennerster begins by reviewing the recent reforms to the National Health Service (NHS) in the UK. Glennerster stresses that these reforms were introduced after the British government had success-fully used global budget constraints to stabilize health care expenditure as a share of Gross Domestic Product (GDP). Thus, the NHS reforms are aimed not at controlling total costs but at improving the efficiency of health care delivery in order to increase patient satisfaction generated by the fixed budget allocated to health.

Glennerster's review of the NHS reforms illuminates the principles underlying the internal market system. The reforms sought to establish markets by separating purchasers from providers, so that buyers and sell-ers of health services could enter into contracts with one another. For example, public hospitals in the UK now compete for contracts from the District Health Authorities (DHAs), who are responsible for purchasing hospital services on behalf of residents of their district. Hospitals also compete for contracts from groups of general practitioners — GP fund-holders — who provide primary care and arrange non-emergency hospi-tal services for their patients.

The NHS markets are "internal" in the sense that buyers and sellers of health care remain within the public sector, where they are subject to global cost constraints set by the government. For example, because DHAs are funded solely by the central government, total DHA purchas-es of hospital services are limited by the amount the government decides to allocate to DHAs.

Rather than reducing costs, as Glennerster emphasizes, the NHS reforms have coincided with the largest increase in NHS spending growth since the 1960s. However, the reforms also show signs of increasing patient satisfaction with the health care system. GP fundholders have had some success negotiating with hospitals for services more in tune with the needs of their patients.

Alan Maynard reviews the NHS reforms in a paper that assesses the case for using market mechanisms to achieve health policy objectives. Maynard identifies three broad policy goals in health care: cost containment, equity and efficiency. Market mechanisms focus on the goal of efficiency. Internal market reforms must be accompanied by government regulation, he writes, to ensure that the pursuit of efficiency does not jeopardize the objectives of cost containment and equity. Maynard is concerned that the NHS reforms have been implemented without an adequate regulatory framework.

Maynard argues that increasing health care efficiency depends on increasing our knowledge about three critical factors. First, how cost effective are medical procedures and technology? Second, what mechanisms can be used to persuade providers to adopt cost-effective practices? And, finally, which institutional framework is best suited to generating information on cost effectiveness and to encouraging providers to change their behaviour in light of that information? Maynard finds that the reforms have not provided an institutional framework for improved efficiency in the NHS.

Clas Rehnberg provides an overview of recent health care reforms in Sweden. Like the UK, Sweden had successfully stabilized health care spending as a percentage of GDP before embarking on market-based reforms. Reforms have been aimed at improving both efficiency and patient satisfaction.

Swedish counties have taken a variety of steps to introduce market mechanisms. Some counties have formed collective purchasing units to represent all patients in a district by contracting with providers for the supply of services. Contracts and performance-based reimbursement are replacing salaries and annual grants. As a result, providers are subject to increased competition, but they also enjoy more autonomy. In addition, the national government has passed legislation designed to increase the freedom of patients to choose their primary care providers.

Rehnberg provides an interesting economic analysis of the Swedish reforms. He discusses the nature of the contracts and the markets for property, capital and labour in the health care sector as well as the potential for market entry and exit. Rehnberg concludes that there are important differences between Sweden's internal health care markets and conventional competitive markets. Sweden has retained public financing of health care, public ownership of health care facilities and central regulation of prices. Rehnberg describes Sweden's internal markets, therefore, as "regulated competition among public providers."

Richard Saltman reviews the reform experience in the UK, Sweden, Finland and Denmark to identify similarities and differences. He finds that internal market reforms in these countries have focussed on how public health care is delivered (the production side) and how revenues are paid to providers (the allocation side). None of these countries has applied the market approach to the financing side of health care. None has sought to create a system in which the amount of care depends largely on ability to pay.

Saltman's international comparison also reveals an interesting paradox. As these countries have introduced internal markets in health care systems, government regulatory responsibilities have not diminished. Instead, governments have recognized the need to regulate internal markets, to ensure that health care standards and guarantees of equal access are maintained.

His comparison allows Saltman to generalize about the tendencies discussed in the preceding papers. He identifies two models of the "purchaser-provider split" in which a purchaser acts as agent for patients: in one model, patients follow the money; in the other, money follows the patients. He also identifies differences in the political accountability of purchasers. Saltman's analysis highlights issues of national as opposed to regional authority over health care, and of different approaches to the same goal: giving people concerned with primary care more control over the purchase of secondary and tertiary care.

Wynand van de Ven and Frederik Schut discuss recent health reforms in the Netherlands. The pre-reform Dutch system combined compulsory public insurance and, for upper-income households, voluntary private insurance for some types of health care ("non-catastrophic" risks). However, private insurers were subject to extensive regulation. Like the Swedish and British reforms, the Dutch reforms were motivated more by efficiency concerns than by cost concerns. Government constraints had already stabilized health care costs as a percentage of GDP.

The authors describe the Dutch reform as a system of regulated competition among both insurers and providers. The government would specify a basic insurance package that would account for 95 percent of health care spending. The formerly private insurers and the sickness funds would compete for the patronage of all individuals. Although maximum provider fees would still be regulated, insurers could individually contract with providers for lower rates or different payment arrangements. Individuals would choose among the insurers' various means of providing the base package. Each insurer would charge a small, fixed premium to each person, who would be free to choose a plan with a lower premium. But by far the largest share of insurers' medical costs would be covered by a risk-adjusted, prospective payment from a central fund, financed largely by payroll-based contributions set by government.

The Dutch reforms were originally scheduled to take four years to implement. Van de Ven and Schut believe full implementation will now take 10 to 15 years. Both the degree of political resistance to the measures and the technical complexity of the proposals were under-estimated when the reform package was launched in 1988. One of the most important technical problems is "cream skimming," or "preferred risk selection." While these authors discuss the particular Dutch experience, in later papers Joshua Wiener and Vivian Hamilton consider this issue further.

MANAGED COMPETITION IN THE UNITED STATES

The section on the European experience is followed by two papers that review the US experience with competing private insurers and providers. The internal market approach to health care reform is closely related to the American theory of "managed competition." If something resembling the Clinton Administration proposals had been adopted, the US system would now be evolving toward an internal market system.

Joshua Wiener reviews managed competition proposals in the US with particular attention to the Clinton Administration's reform proposal. While these proposals were promoted as a non-governmental, market-driven set of institutions, their details made clear the need for a large government bureaucracy with extensive powers. One reason for regulation, as also discussed in the chapter by van de Ven and Schut and the chapter by Hamilton, was to prevent risk selection from undermining fair price competition. Another concern was the need for complex enrolment arrangements and for subsidized private insurance premiums for low-income households.

These and other difficulties required institutions, the Clinton "health alliances," that were in turn attacked as large new bureaucracies. But the concerns to which the regulations were meant to respond are very real, and Wiener cautions that market mechanisms would have to be introduced very carefully to ensure that the objectives of global cost containment, equity and consumer choice would not be sacrificed. This dilemma, the contrast between the need for regulation and the rhetoric of competition, helped defeat the Clinton reform effort.

Joseph White discusses the "management" side of managed competition, assessing how well care might be managed in the US and, by extension, elsewhere. He divides American managed care into three models: third-party management, the traditional group- or staff-model HMO and the risk-bearing gatekeeper model. (In actual marketing, many different systems are called HMOs.)

Third-party management of providers by private insurers depends on effective enforcement of treatment guidelines. Studies show that effective third-party management can reduce health care costs slightly. But guidelines are difficult to develop and implement everywhere, and the US system of competing insurance plans poses special problems.

The group- or staff-model HMO has a better record of cost control than pure third-party managed care. Individuals (or employers) contract with a group of physicians for all care; the latter may establish more conservative practice norms, but, with less rigid rules, make exceptions when necessary. Yet White argues that these systems cannot expand quickly, nor cover the entire US population.

In the risk-bearing gatekeeper model, a primary care physician or group has financial responsibility for managing care in order to reduce total costs — in essence, by limiting the number of referrals and prescriptions. The savings of this form of managed care can approach those of traditional HMOs, but in the American circumstance of multiple insurers and multiple physician affiliations the risk-bearing gatekeeper model also puts physicians at great and arguably arbitrary financial risk.

While all three managed care models can reduce costs relative to fee-for-service payment systems with no management controls, even the "best case" estimates of potential cost savings are not dramatic. White concludes that the US has more to learn from other countries' methods of imposing global cost constraints than other countries have to learn from US models of managed care.

The Potential for Internal Market Reforms in Canada

The volume is completed by four Canadian perspectives on the internal market concept.

Vivian Hamilton considers the risk selection problem. If private or public payments to insurance funds do not adequately reflect observable patient characteristics associated with high health costs (such as age, sex and previous health record), funds have incentives to target low-risk, low-cost customers and avoid high-risk, high-cost members. While most studies have applied to competition among private insurers, the same incentives may act on competing providers of care within publicly financed health care systems, such as the British GP fundholders.

Proposed remedies range from better demographic estimators to reinsurance pools for some conditions to risk adjustments based on actual claims experience — all with their own difficulties. Although van de Ven and Schut believe a solution can be developed, the Dutch have not yet done so. Hamilton provides a thorough assessment of the current alternatives.

The next two papers present concrete proposals for implementing internal markets in Canada.

Åke Blomqvist places internal market proposals in a historical context. In the first wave of health care reform, Canada and most European countries established universal access to publicly financed health care. Public health care systems are now engaged in a second wave of reform in which the concerns are cost control and efficiency. Blomqvist believes that internal markets can help to achieve these second-wave objectives.

European reforms provide models for introducing internal markets in Canada. Contracts awarded on a competitive basis by regional boards that purchase services from public hospitals could increase the efficiency of the hospital system. Similar gains could be generated by moving away from the current Canadian practice of paying primary care physicians on a fee-for-service basis. Instead, physicians could be paid on a capitation (or per patient) basis and could be made financially responsible for part of their patients' total costs, including drugs and some hospital services.

Monique Jérôme-Forget and Claude Forget argue that cost control is particularly important in Canada in light of the fiscal problems facing Canadian governments. They observe that reform will work best if it builds on the strengths of the existing system. Therefore, they argue for taking advantage of the professional and ethical values that are part of the training and practice culture of physicians. The authors would put those values to the service of a form of entrepreneurship that could guarantee quality within constraints.

Their internal market proposal focusses on the creation of Targeted Medical Agencies (TMAs), groups of up to 30 physicians responsible for managing medical and hospital care on behalf of their patients. Patients would register with TMAs, which would be paid by government on a per-patient basis instead of under the current fee-for-service system. Payment rates would vary according to type of patient, to allow for the fact that certain patient characteristics (age, sex, pre-existing medical problems) are associated with higher medical costs. Instead of receiving fixed annual grants from government, hospitals would be paid by TMAs. TMAs could contract with each other — for example, a TMA made up of GPs could arrange to purchase services from one made up of specialists.

This proposal would establish market incentives for physicians to manage care effectively on behalf of their patients, while preserving government's role of financing health care and setting an overall limit on public health care spending.

In the final paper, Robert Evans comments on the potential for internal markets in Canada. He views internal markets as a tool for improving health care management, but warns that designing internal markets with effective incentives will be difficult. A long period of consensus-building will be necessary before the major changes required to establish internal markets can be implemented. In the meantime, there is a danger that the health reform agenda will be captured by proponents of what Evans calls "parallel markets" (private health care) or "marginal markets" (user fees), both of which would likely increase total costs without improving efficiency. Evans proposes a strategy of "piecemeal, carefully targeted, and carefully thought-out changes in incentives," which could be implemented without the broad degree of support needed for major reforms.

CONCLUSION

As should be evident even from this introduction, the authors in this volume bring a wide array of perspectives and opinions to bear on both experience with and prospects for internal markets. For example, Glennerster and Maynard reach two different conclusions after reviewing the same experience, the British NHS reforms. Glennerster believes that the reforms have been a useful step forward, while Maynard finds them to be mostly misconceived. The whole idea of an internal market can vary according to the standpoint of the country. In Sweden, it can be seen as serving to expand choice. In the US, the most controversial element might be imposing a budget.

Whatever the context and whatever the specific proposal, this book makes clear that internal market approaches will be a part of the international health care agenda for some time. They have been implemented partially, mainly in northern Europe, as modifications to systems in which governments provided health services directly, rather than insured private care. Yet one can imagine any system evolving in this direction. Therefore, both the logic and the implementation of internal markets should be considered carefully.

Both experience and thought experiments, as described in these papers, suggest that a lot can go wrong with poorly designed internal market proposals. But no country is in a position to smugly believe that its current arrangements are ideal. Even if existing approaches are desirable, a nation like Canada may have reason to fear that they cannot be maintained.

Nations are usually reluctant to embark on major reforms, and some countries have much greater problems than others. But policy makers in every country must think hard about their alternatives. We hope that this book contributes to a practical discussion of whether and how internal market arrangements can guarantee equal access to health care and can control costs in a manner that will increase the value that societies receive in return for their huge expenditures on health care.

H O W A R D   G L E N N E R S T E R

INTERNAL MARKETS:

CONTEXT AND STRUCTURE

The oil shocks of the 1970s and their aftermath checked the almost continuous growth of State welfare that had occurred since the second world war in most advanced economies. For 30 years virtually all western countries had expanded the share of their national incomes devoted to social programmes. From the mid-1970s this trend was checked most sharply in the United Kingdom. The share of GDP devoted to social spending in the UK stayed constant for more than a decade and a half, from 1975 to 1991. Since social security spending rose as unemployment rose, the pressure on health and other programmes was intense. Initially, the changed economic climate did not produce structural change. For a decade or more, governments followed a policy of belt tightening rather than radical reform. Eventually, some governments found that path unsustainable, and the UK in particular took dramatic measures.

Since health expenditure in the UK is financed and controlled by the central exchequer it has been possible to set firm budget ceilings to health spending for a long period. During the early years of the Thatcher Administration health spending in the UK rose more slowly in real terms than the age-weighted population. Per capita spending on health, adjusted for age, thus fell in the mid-1980s.[1] This provoked a series of scandals, with children in need of intensive care being unable to gain access to hospital among other embarrassments. In the UK political context such harsh rationing decisions tend to land at the door of the national politicians who carry the blame. Prime Minister Thatcher was not amused and called for a radical review of the financing of the National Health Service (NHS).

It is important that overseas observers appreciate this sequence of events. The UK health reforms were not concerned with halting the rise in health costs. Cost control had already been achieved. Rather, the reforms were aimed at coping with the consequences of imposing limits to the growth in health spending.

Some in government began with the idea that it would be possible to privatize parts of the service and expand the private health insurance sector. This line of reform was opposed by none other than the Conservative Chancellor, Nigel Lawson.[2] He and the Treasury were convinced that it would be foolish to give up the tight control on spending the UK system already provided and that private health insurance markets did not produce efficient outcomes.

The government's reform white paper[3] began with an affirmation of the principles that underlay the old NHS — free access by the whole population to health care, financed from general taxation. Within those constraints the government was searching for ways in which to get more out of the hospitals and family doctors for the same expenditure.

Fiscal constraint was only one force at work. Increasingly the old structures, dating back to the immediate post-war period, were beginning to show their age. Universal services run by a single bureaucratic agency gave the promise of equal treatment and equal access. This was rarely achieved. Achieved or not, it tended to be at the cost of consumer choice, which was becoming wider in the growing private service sector. The capacity to shop around in housing, insurance, financial services, and supermarkets increasingly contrasted favourably with take-it-or-leave-it attitudes in public services.

The powerlessness of consumers, their inability to take their custom elsewhere, to use the sanction of "exit," meant that social services gradually became complacent and unresponsive. Power shifted to the professionals who controlled the services. Structures evolved that enhanced their working conditions, not the users' satisfaction. This was a gradual but insidious process. In the 1960s and 1970s attempts were made to increase users' influence through various kinds of consumer participation schemes or through enhanced complaints procedures. Neither method proved entirely satisfactory, least of all in the health services.

In the 1980s economic liberalism began to grow in appeal for just these reasons. The collapse of the command economies in Eastern Europe had a profound impact on the climate of ideas about forms of welfare. In its radical form the new economic liberalism would have abolished the State welfare institutions of the post-war period. Yet, despite people's frustrations with these institutions, support for their original goals remained strong in many countries, especially in Britain, and especially for the NHS. For this reason, the NHS reforms in the UK present a paradigm, though the same forces were evident in the case of other Northern European health care systems and in other public services throughout the OECD area.[4]

The double forces at work behind health care and other welfare reforms were, therefore, budget constraints forced by fiscal pressures and a growing consumerism. What emerged from this climate was an apparently magical formula — the view that it was possible to increase consumer satisfaction and the efficiency of these services, while keeping the principle of free and equal access at no more cost. What politician could resist?

A New Approach

This new strategy involved keeping tax-based finance but introducing an element of competition among public providers. It has been variously labelled as the introduction of "quasi markets"[5] or "market-type mechanisms"[6] or "planned markets."[7] In the United States the approach is invested with a more appealing title — "reinventing government."[8] Nowhere has this approach been more widely adopted than in the field of health care, where both the fiscal constraints and the deficiencies of monopolistic social agencies had become most evident.

The extent of the competitive dose has, however, varied. One version confines the competition to suppliers of services. A public authority purchases services on behalf of its entire population. Monopoly remains on the demand side. Consumers, as individuals, have no greater choice. They may gain cheaper or better services but only if the purchaser fully reflects their preferences.

A second version takes the competitive logic further. Individuals ought to be able to choose which purchaser they will patronize. It is only this more extreme model, which fully meets the urge to make the consumer king, that motivated many reformers. It is the model of the Health Maintenance Organization (HMO) in the US whereby members join and pay a premium, and the HMO buys hospital and other care for them. We find examples of both kinds of competition in Western health care reforms — supply-side only and both supply- and demand-side competition. The fullest version of all is to give vouchers to consumers themselves or to their parents or guardians — the school voucher and the UK education reforms are an example of this approach.

Saltman and von Otter[9] have charted the way in which public health care systems in Scandinavia, Eastern Europe and the UK have moved in similar directions, introducing an element of competition among public providers. Local agencies of the State retained the duty to ensure that their populations had universal access to health care, and they chose among competing hospitals or other public providers to supply services for these populations. The county councils in Sweden and the municipalities in Finland are beginning to do this. Saltman and von Otter argue that the combination of needs-based purchasing power with decentralized consumer choice enhances the modern polity, creating what they call a "civil democracy."

In the Netherlands the aim is to combine universal access with the right of the Dutch citizen to choose among alternative health insurance agencies. Similar ideas lie behind President Clinton's reform package.

The British reforms, unusually, embody elements of both these alternative models of competition. District Health Authorities purchase most services on behalf of their whole populations. They choose among competing public hospitals. GP fundholders purchase non-emergency care for their patients in the way that an HMO does. Patients can choose their GP and therefore their purchaser. Social service departments purchase long-term care for their whole communities from a range of public and private providers.

These changes to NHS and other British social services, like other reforms in Europe, challenge the old command-and-control paradigm of social welfare. They decentralize purchasing power without going the whole way to a private consumer market. Yet consumer choice and competition carry dangers as well as advantages. There are difficult tradeoffs to be made between improving efficiency and ensuring fairness, between the capacity to plan and the scope for innovation.[10]

THE NHS INTERNAL MARKETS

A brief examination of the NHS reforms introduced in 1991 serves to illustrate the hopes and problems involved in "planning" health care markets.

Two principles of internal market reform had been in competition since 1986. One derived from the ideas of Alain Enthoven, though adapted by NHS managers. The central idea was to split the finance of health care from the function of providing it, as happens in so many other health care systems. But the aim was also to keep the single purchaser and planning function intact. District Health Authorities would continue to be financed by the central government, receiving a sum of money that reflected the size, age structure and health status of their populations. They would then contract with hospitals in their area or beyond it to provide the full range of services they could afford with their budget. The hospitals would become independent entities no longer administered by the districts. They would have to win contracts and revenue or go bust. Such, at least, was the theory.

The advantage of such an arrangement was seen to be that it combined the capacity for districts to plan services for their whole area with the power to threaten a poorly performing hospital with loss of its contract. Exit power would be exercised in a collective way. Critics argued that this model gave little extra power or choice to consumers. No patient could change his or her purchaser if they were dissatisfied unless they moved house to another district. As has become evident since, large-scale monopoly purchasers like districts, purchasing for 250,000 and more patients, tend to make cosy relationships with the large local providers. They are very dependent on the providers for their expert medical knowledge.

Competing with this model was a very different one. It had much smaller purchasers — the family doctor — acting on behalf of the patient. The idea of giving general practitioners the capacity to buy hospital services on behalf of their patients predated the Conservative government's white paper.

The principle had been discussed by Alan Maynard, Professor of Health Economics at York University, in the early 1980s.[11] Patients lacked the knowledge to be informed purchasers of health care on their own. They were reliant on professional advisers to tell them whether they needed a service and from whom to get it. In the NHS, GPs are those advisers. Why not give them the task of buying services on behalf of their patients? This would combine consumer choice and competition between GPs and hospitals for the patient's custom. It shared many characteristics with the American HMO model.

Transporting the HMO model to the UK posed real difficulties. There was simply no comparably large primary care organization. Most HMOs are very large by the standard of British general practice. Many are as large as a District Health Authority, some larger. American experience suggested that small HMOs were financially vulnerable. An unfortunately large number of expensive patients needing emergency treatment in any one year could bankrupt a small HMO. To average out this possibility the "risk pool" needs to be large. The American work suggested that HMOs were at risk if their patient list was smaller than 50,000 or so.[12] No UK practice came anywhere near that size. Only about 40 percent of practices had more than 7,000 patients.

Other research in the US suggested that the flat-rate premium produced other problems. Some patients cost a lot more than others and could be predicted to cost more. For that reason doctors were reluctant to take them onto their books — a process called "biased selection" or "cream skimming."

Those in the Department of Health working on the reforms were well aware of these problems and attempted to build into the scheme a set of safeguards. First, the scheme was to be confined to large practices. The white paper said the scheme would apply to practices with "at least 11,000 patients." This limit was lowered to 9,000 in 1990 and to 7,000 in 1992.

Secondly, the budget was to cover only non-emergency care. Most of the treatments the GP could buy from the hospital were standard, relatively inexpensive procedures. The budget would exclude any open-ended treatment that might result from a GP's referral for a simple case. The white paper said the services GPs could buy would include all out-patient care, diagnostic tests and a restricted range of inpatient and day-case treatments "such as hip replacements and cataract removals, for which there may be some choice over time and place of treatment." It was not until much later that the Department of Health worked out a full list of treatments covered by the scheme.

This constriction of Maynard's vision of a much fuller internal market illustrates problems involved in the practical implementation of a quasi-market reform. These complications were particularly pronounced in the British case because there were, at the time, few lessons to be learned from other countries. The origins of the fundholding scheme were, therefore, varied, but they did focus on some key deficiencies of the old NHS. GP fundholding also went furthest toward the notion of opening up the service to competition and transferring purchasing power from State bureaucracies to nearer the patient.

REFORM TO WHAT END?

It is too early to come to definitive judgements about the reforms, but the early results suggest that it is this more thorough-going application of the internal market model that has had the most impact.[13] What they have not done is reduce costs. On the contrary, the introduction of market-based reforms was accompanied by the fastest increase in spending on the NHS since the 1960s. Cost reduction, however, was not the intent of these reforms. The goal was to improve standards and consumer responsiveness. Fierce cost cutting had already been achieved in previous budgets, and these new reforms were introduced in part to deal with the after-effects of those cuts.

The government working paper that launched much of these changes was entitled *Working for Patients*. This emphasis is well suited to the theoretical underpinnings of the "internal" market concept and the public policy realities that allowed these ideas to reach implementation. The seductions of a scheme under which consumers could signal dissatisfaction with "exit" within a system that maintained universality through wholly public expenditure were what drew politicians to this option in the first place. The fact that the system was greatly modified to deal with potential problems (i.e., insurable practice sizes, cream skimming, etc.) reflects issues both of implementation and of bureaucratic momentum. It does not, however, limit our ability to judge whether this manifestation of the internal market idea has met with concrete success. In this respect, we are constrained by the relatively recent enactment of these policies, but preliminary conclusions are possible.

The promise of an internal market in health care was largely one of increased consumer power. At this early stage the results are necessarily tentative, but leading indicators do seem to show that increased consumer power is happening. In a fairly exhaustive treatment of the results of the fundholding system (as distinct from the District Health Authority reforms) by Glennerster, Matsaganis, and Owens,[14] the ability of fundholding practitioners to exact changes in the quality and method of delivery of services to their patients is apparent. Hospitals have grown more responsive to their demands. The choice of higher-level provision is beginning to be allocated on the basis of efficiency. Fundholders' drug prescriptions have been reduced *vis-à-vis* those of non-fundholders.

The track record of the UK is therefore mixed. The original aim of the internal market — to improve the system at no greater cost — has not been universally successful. The improvements thus far, however, hold out the promise that the concept of separating the purchaser from the provider and then giving each the right incentives to deliver high-quality health care in an efficient, patient-centred way, is producing results. It is far less clear in the parallel reforms to social care. Implementation and the right mix of incentives are critical.

1. H. Glennerster and M. Matsaganis, "The English and Swedish Health Care Reforms," *International Journal of Health Services,* Vol. 24, no. 2 (1994), pp. 231–51.
2. N. Lawson, *The View from No. 11: Memoirs of a Tory Radical* (London: Bantam Press, 1992).
3. Department of Health, *Working for Patients* (London: HMSO, 1989).
4. Organisation for Economic Co-operation and Development, *Progress in Structural Reform: An Overview* (Paris: OECD, 1992).
5. J. Le Grand and W. Bartlett, *Quasi-Markets and Social Policy* (London: Macmillan, 1993).
6. OECD Occasional Papers, Market-Type Mechanisms Series, OECD, Paris, 1992–93.
7. Richard B. Saltman and Casten von Otter, *Planned Markets and Public Competition: Stragetic Reform in Northern European Health Systems* (Milton Keynes: Open University Press, 1992).
8. David Osborne and Ted Gaebler, *Reinventing Government: How the Entrepreneurial Spirit is Transforming the Public Sector* (Reading, Mass.: Addison-Wesley, 1992).
9. Saltman and von Otter, *Planned Markets and Public Competition.*
10. R. Robinson and J. Le Grand (eds.), *Evaluating the NHS Reforms* (London: King's Fund Institute, 1994).
11. Alan Maynard, "Performance Incentives," in Teeling G. Smith (ed.), *Education and General Practice* (London: Office of Health Economics, 1986).
12. J. Wiener and P. Ferris, *GP Budget Holding in the UK: Lessons from America* (London: King's Fund Institute, 1990).
13. Robinson and Le Grand, *Evaluating the NHS Reforms.*
14. H. Glennerster, M. Matsaganis and P. Owens, *Wild Card or Winning Hand? Implementing Fundholding* (Milton Keynes: Open University Press, 1994).

A L A N   M A Y N A R D

INTERNAL MARKETS AND HEALTH CARE:

A BRITISH PERSPECTIVE

INTRODUCTION

Why use the market mechanism in health care systems? Policy-makers seek three goals when reforming these systems: cost containment, equity and efficiency. The potential use of markets as a means of achieving cost control is much discussed in theory but shows little evidence of effectiveness in practice. The practice of cost control, which depends on a global budget and what Reinhardt[1] calls the "single pipe" funding system, appears to have had some success in Britain, Germany, New Zealand and the Scandinavian countries. Governments in these countries have adopted market mechanisms to facilitate the achievement of neither cost containment nor equity, an objective which again is quite well served in these systems, but improved efficiency of resource allocation — i.e., to ensure that costs are minimized and health benefits are maximized. They are discovering that the simple-minded prioritization and pursuit of one goal (efficiency) affects the attainment of other goals (cost containment and equity). The recognition of these interdependencies is affecting the design and implementation of market reforms.

In the United States, it seems that the ideological battle between left and right has created confusion about means and ends. Such confusion is the essence of politics in Europe and Australasia also. The egalitarians attack the actual deficiencies of the market mechanism in delivering and funding care, and advocate their collective ideal. The libertarians attack the actual deficiencies of collective health care systems, and advocate *their* ideal (the market). The nature of the competing "ideals" and "actuals" is described in the appendix.[2]

The characteristics of this "split personality" approach to the debate about health care policy are familiar. They facilitate the adoption of imperfectly designed and executed reforms, as in Britain since 1989. As a result, policy making is not informed by evidence and clinical practice is not evidence-based — because the debate is dominated by rhetoric rather than knowledge about the cost effectiveness of policy options.

In the first section of this paper the objectives of policy makers are discussed and the nature of health care markets is explored. In the second section the tradeoffs among cost containment, equity and efficiency are examined briefly. It is argued that mechanisms intended to achieve cost containment and equity, involving substantial government intervention, are well identified, and that the political protagonists and their policy analysts should not confuse the policy debate on the potential of market mechanisms to reach these goals. Instead, they should focus on how markets and rival means of achieving greater efficiency in resource allocation, within a regime of global budgets, single-source finance and access determined by the patient's capacity to benefit from care, can be evaluated.

POLICY OBJECTIVES AND THE DESIGN AND PERFORMANCE OF HEALTH CARE MARKETS

Policy Objectives

In addition to the pursuit of cost containment and equity, there is much discussion of the "rules" that should be used to determine access to health care.[3] In systems based on egalitarian values, access is determined largely by "need." However, need is usually badly defined by legislators in these systems and it clearly could be both a demand and a supply concept.[4] It is assumed here that the appropriate definition of need, in an egalitarian system, is capacity to benefit per unit of cost — i.e., in such systems, access to health care should be determined by the patient's ability to benefit (the benefit principle).

An alternative (libertarian) access rule is willingness and ability to pay. This principle is dominant in many markets for goods and services but has generally been abandoned in health care markets (even that of the US, where 50 cents of the health care dollar are "socialized"). The abandonment of this principle is a product of market failures that have proved impossible to remedy in practice but that are still deemed soluble by market-oriented reformers who believe that their designs, like Christianity, have not failed but have yet to be tried!

The implication of the abandonment of the willingness-and-ability-to-pay allocation rule, and the adoption of the benefit principle, is that two judgements have to be made.

1. Which health care interventions are cost effective? If scarce resources are to be allocated to maximize benefits (measured in terms of enhancement of length and quality of life) derived from limited budgets, then rules of "appropriateness" and "practice guidelines," informed by the knowledge base of cost effectiveness, must be created and used to "ration" resources.

2. How much will government spend to buy marginal increases in health gain (or quality adjusted life years — QALYs)? With no market signals to inform funding decisions, judgements based on social, economic, technical and political criteria are unavoidable.

In a system where access to health care is determined by capacity to benefit per unit of cost, the potential outcome is efficient and ethical (in that there is no inefficiency and consequently potential patients are not deprived of health care from which they could benefit). Such a system is potentially inequitable if the distribution of capacity to benefit is unequal, as it usually is between rich and poor. The system may be equal in terms of access but not in terms of treatment and health outcome.

The adoption of the benefit principle together with "single pipe" funding of a global budget may produce efficiency, cost containment and equal access in principle. All health care funding, public and private, comes from one source: households. Households pay for health care by either taxes to the State, premiums to insurers or directly (e.g., co-payments). Where funding is fragmented (such as coming from all three sources), attempts to control one "pipe" usually create increased funding flows in the other pipes, with little overall control of total expenditure. If funding is from one source, such as the State, cost control cannot be circumvented so easily, and typically it seems that systems with single-pipe funding manage to control expenditure more effectively.

Cost control is difficult because most health care interventions are unproven, and much, or even most, resource allocation is driven by provider rhetoric and self-interest (i.e., by provider capture) rather than by science-based knowledge about "what works." These inefficiencies have increasingly attracted the attention of policy makers in the last decade, 20 years after the research literature clearly identified the problem.[5]

It is now recognized that ignorance about the cost-effectiveness of competing therapies means that many clinical choices are made in circumstances of great uncertainty, and that one of the results of this is apparently wide variations in clinical practice, adjusted for age and sex.[6] In addition, there is evidence of considerable inappropriate practice,[7] with too many ineffective interventions and not enough effective care.[8]

Thus the pursuit of efficiency has been unsuccessful in all health care systems. It is concern about deficiencies in the system of resource allocation that has induced policy makers to opt for reforms that are poorly targeted, are not evidence-based, and may reverse gains in cost control and equity.

The Market "Solution"

A market is a network of buyers and sellers. Market-orientated ideologues advocate "free" markets, but always and everywhere public and private decision-makers regulate the market to serve their own ends (i.e., they formally and informally seek to control prices, quantities and quality). Capitalists are the enemies of capitalism: they constrain the flexible functioning of markets to increase their profits. Adam Smith predicted "conspiracy" in product markets where entrepreneurs have considerable market power (e.g., in pharmaceutical markets today).

> People of the same trade rarely meet together, even for merriment and diversion, but the conversation ends in a conspiracy against the public or in some contrivance to raise prices.[9]

Labour unions, such as those of physicians, also regulate markets to serve their needs, as Adam Smith argued:

> The pretence that corporations are necessary for the better government of the trade, is without any foundation. The real and effectual discipline which is exercised over a workman, is not

that of his corporation, but that of his customers. It is the fear of losing their employment which restrains his frauds and corrects his negligence.[10]

Markets are always and everywhere regulated by private and public agencies anxious to control the prices, quantities and quality of the goods and services traded. The policy problem is how to control these regulators so that their activities serve the interests of consumers rather than the producers.

The Chicago economist and Nobel laureate Ronald Coase described the inevitability of such market regulation very nicely when discussing the functioning of the market for stocks and shares and primary commodities:

It is not without significance that these exchanges, often used by economists as examples of a perfect market and perfect competition, are markets in which transactions are highly regulated (and this quite apart from any government regulation that there may be). It suggests, I think correctly, that for anything approaching perfect competition to exist, an intricate system of rules and regulations would normally be needed.[11]

Market reform in health care systems takes two forms. The attempt to create competition on both the supply and demand sides of the market is generally referred to as "managed competition," and one of its prime initiators over the last 15 or more years is Alain Enthoven.[12] Enthoven proposes competition among highly regulated insurance funders and providers, with the regulation required to create and sustain competition. The British health care reforms have involved a limited form of managed care. These reforms have left funding arrangements in place — a tax-financed (single-pipe) global budget — and have addressed only the challenges of creating market competition in the supply of health care: the internal market or regulated competition.

Whether the desire is to devise managed competition or an internal market, such mechanisms can be created only by extensive regulation of the networks of purchasers and providers (i.e., the market). This is well described at the level of principle by the Jackson Hole proposals[13] and in their subsequent elaboration.[14]

The British internal market proposals have been inadequately articulated in that either there is no regulatory framework or the regulatory framework is inadequately designed.[15] Britain, like any nation adopting more explicit market mechanisms, must create rules about price setting, capital allocation and labour markets that are consistent with policy goals. This is not an easy task.

1. *Pricing Rules.* The British government has required providers to fix prices (P) equal to average costs (AC). Even if providers had any idea about the nature of their cost structure (which they do not!), such a pricing rule would be unlikely to produce efficiency in resource use. Typically in markets where there are many buyers and relatively few sellers (e.g., food retailing), prices tend to be fixed. In markets where there are few buyers and sellers (i.e., in many or even most health care markets), posted prices tend to be an invitation to negotiate. Those who buy in bulk and over long periods will typically get lower prices than those who buy the same service in small quantities on a "spot market." Knowledge about the nature and availability of bulk discounts will be covert and buyers will have to search and negotiate skilfully.

Setting a pricing rule (P = AC) is at best an expedient to enhance the skills of finance directors in setting costs and producing price data to facilitate market trading and contract shifting. Such a Stalinist approach has little logic in the medium term if the objective of the reforms is indeed to decentralize decision making, encourage entrepreneurial behaviour and improve resource allocation.

However, the risk inherent in such trading practices, particularly in a market where there are risks of quality competition, is that price flexibility will lead to cost inflation. Conservative pricing rules (P = AC), if they can be enforced by the market regulator, may facilitate cost control even if their effects on efficiency may be perverse.

2. *Capital Market Rules.* The British government has been reluctant to permit National Health Service (NHS) Trust hospitals and other State providers to have access to the capital market. Instead, whilst capital is now "priced" in that providers have to pay a six percent rate of return, the stock remains poor and the total level of investment is determined in total by government fiat and prioritized with investment appraisal techniques.

Britain may follow the New Zealand route and permit State hospitals to borrow in the private capital market. Provided the hospitals can provide collateral and assured revenue flows, the banks will lend. But this requires the sale of the hospitals and/or clear assurances from the

State about their funding intentions. The logic of unleashing forces such as this is the privatization of the hospital stock. This is not without its risks: again, quality competition and duplication of plant and equipment may emerge. This may produce cost inflation and pressure on public funds, which governments may be unable or unwilling to meet, unless it favours tacitly the privatization of health care finance. If funding deficiencies emerged, it is likely that private insurance would increase and the system would move from single-pipe to "dual-pipe" funding. The great merit of single-pipe funding is that efforts to control finance are easier to manage. If dual- or multiple-funding mechanisms arose, attempts to control, for instance, public funding, would, if successful, lead to expansion in the size of another (e.g., private) pipe and abandonment of the benefit principle. Relaxation of existing capital controls that create inefficient resource allocation could facilitate increased cost inflation.

3. *Labour Market Rules.* The rhetoric of reformers advocating managed competition and regulated competition (internal market) favours decentralized decision-making on skill mix, labour rewards and employment contracts and asserts that the resource savings may be considerable.

This hypothesis may be tenable in a service industry constrained by remarkable labour market restrictions devised by the professions and trade unions and condoned by government for reasons of political support. However, once again such a reform may be double-edged. In egalitarian motivated and designed systems such as the British NHS, the remuneration and numbers of professionals such as doctors are centrally controlled. Five years after announcement of the NHS reforms, few NHS employers have changed — this even though, in principle, they are free to do so within the constraints of cash-limited NHS funding.

Why have they behaved in this manner? One explanation is that the old-style NHS contract for life for NHS consultants and general practitioners benefits their employers. They have a guaranteed supply of labour and, whilst employers carry the risk of having over-capacity if revenues fall, the price they pay for labour services is relatively low. If employees had short-term contracts, the risks to them of fluctuating demand and redundancy would be greater and they would expect higher levels of pay.

Thus "freeing up" wage bargaining may be costly. If carried out at the local level, transaction costs would be higher than with national pay bargaining, and levels of remuneration would probably rise. Whether the gains from improved resource allocation with short-term contracts would exceed these costs is an empirical issue.

The maintenance of manpower planning within the new NHS internal market is incongruous.[16] However, for those policy-makers in the Treasury it has the attraction of complementing rigidities in the pay of clinicians by controlling doctors' numbers and, hence, constraining an important element in the health care system: physician-induced demand and the associated inflation.

4. *Behaviour and Incentives.* The ideology of the 1980s, with Reagan and Thatcher advocating the creation of markets to replace the public sector, was a crude one. Occasionally their policy analysts supported this advocacy by quoting Adam Smith:

> It is not from the benevolence of the butcher, the brewer and the baker, that we expect our dinner, but from their regard to their own interest. We address ourselves, not to their humanity but to their self-love, and never talk to them of our necessities but to their advantages.[17]

This stereotype of vigorous competition, "red in tooth and claw," rarely exists in most markets. Indeed Adam Smith argued that self-regulation rather than the pressures created by self-interest in competitive markets was the more usual and most effective form of controlling the behaviour of purchasers and providers.

> Those general rules of conduct when they have been fixed in our mind by habitual reflection, are of great use in correcting the misrepresentations of self-love concerning what is fit and proper to be done in our particular situation...The regard of those general rules of conduct, is what is properly called a sense of duty, a principle of greatest consequence in human life, and the only principle by which the bulk of mankind are capable of directing their actions.[18]

In the US, Relman[19] and Fuchs[20] have argued that the commercialization of medicine poses major ethical threats: if doctors own facilities, for example, they may create unnecessary demand for patient care and income for their bank accounts. Professional control of practice, the exercise of Smith's sense of duty, has failed; and perhaps this is not surprising given that medical codes such as the Hippocratic oath often appear to be about cartelization and income generation for professions as much as about serving the interests of the patient.[21]

If these professional cartels could be reformed and a sense of duty used to create a knowledge-based Hippocratic oath with explicit performance criteria, the medical profession might be able to heal itself! Whether it could do so effectively at a cost less than that imposed by the internal market is again an empirical issue.

5. *Resource Allocation Principles.* Whether reform managed competition as in the Netherlands or regulated competition as in England, equity in resource allocation is an important policy issue. If insurers are to compete, their income has to be risk adjusted by appropriate regulatory intervention. If non-competing NHS purchasers are to buy health care from competing suppliers in the UK, their funding has to be based on weighted capitation that reflects need. Such regulatory interventions create a "level playing field" for competition and facilitate equity in access for those countries adhering to the benefit principle.

Whether equity in access to health care (i.e., needs-based funding or resource allocation) leads to equity in health is an empirical matter. Much health care expenditure appears to have little impact on health, although patient and carer utility may be derived from the care processes even if health gains are meagre.

Overview

Markets are always regulated, and policy makers have to be clear, when establishing these mechanisms, about their objectives. With objectives identified, the issues of importance are whether in theory and in practice the development of market mechanisms facilitates their achievement better than do existing or some other set of arrangements.

The market reforms in health care systems worldwide have been implemented with poor definition of policy objectives. In particular, the focus on efficiency has often ignored the equity and cost containment goals and the unavoidable tradeoff inherent in reordering these priorities. In some cases this lack of focus may be part of a deliberate political agenda driven by ideology (but perhaps not given the short time horizon of politicians!).

The reforms have also been driven with a nice failure to review evidence on the effectiveness of health care market reforms. The evidence, such as it is, is not compelling after more than a decade of managed competition in places such as the US.[22] The unwillingness of some reformers (e.g., the British) to add to this stock of knowledge by evaluating their radical reforms is depressing and leaves everyone poorly informed after three years of market reform.[23]

USING MARKET MECHANISMS IN THE HEALTH CARE MARKET

Introduction

Given the characteristics of the health care market, in particular moral hazard, physician-induced demand and the unproven nature of most interventions, the primary policy objective is cost containment. This is best achieved by global budgets, perhaps complemented by incentive structures that reward providers who do "less" and penalize those who do "more."

With cost inflation contained, the policy issues are equity and efficiency. Allocation of resources on the basis of ability to benefit at the margin can provide equality of access, but it will not necessarily provide equality of treatment or outcome (i.e., health). Using the health care system to equalize the distribution of health status is probably inefficient; a more productive route may be better education, improved housing and the reduction of poverty. However, the cost effectiveness of such policies is not well established and some of these interventions would violate libertarian ideals and be seen as very costly by some parts of society.

If the equity and cost containment issues are well addressed by relatively proven and explicit policy instruments, the issue is how to improve the efficiency of resource allocation. Three issues have to be addressed in any discussion of efficiency:

1. What works? That is, what is the cost effectiveness of interventions in health care and health promotion?

2. How can we change provider behaviour? That is, what is the cost effectiveness of monetary and non-monetary interventions, or, as Lomas nicely summarized it, "How do you teach old (and not so old) docs new tricks?"[24]

3. What is the appropriate institutional framework in which to facil-

itate the application of knowledge about the cost effectiveness of technologies and behaviours?

Technology Assessment

Not only is the knowledge base in medicine threadbare, there are also significant problems in remedying this situation. A major motive behind clinical and economic evaluation appears to be not enhancement of the knowledge base, but development of curriculum vitae and career prospects.[25] Deficiencies in statistical and other aspects of refereeing result in poor studies being published in apparently good, refereed journals. As a consequence the knowledge base is corrupted.[26]

Such deficiencies in the system of creating knowledge are well known. Nearly 20 years ago Bailar[27] argued that there were more quacks in statistics than in medicine and that "there may be a greater danger to public welfare from statistical dishonesty than from almost any other form of dishonesty." Despite these arguments, poor clinical science continues to be a problem, compounded often by economists' uncritical use of clinical data in economic evaluations.[28] Evaluation of the cost effectiveness of health promotion is very poor and health initiatives are usually driven by prayer rather than science.[29]

With deficiencies in the volume and quality of evaluations, the creation of practice guidelines and appropriateness criteria must be a tentative enterprise. When a biased and poor science base is mixed with the opinions and judgements of "experts" and "consensus groups," the argument of Marx:

> The secret of life is honesty and fair play. If you can fake that, you've made it. — Groucho Marx

should be countervailed by the views of Mao:

> Knowledge is a matter of science, and no dishonesty or conceit whatsoever is permissible. What is required is definitely the reverse: honesty and modesty. — Mao Tse-Tung

Honesty and modesty must be to the fore!

Behaviour Change

If existing knowledge were synthesized to identify what is known and what is unknown, the policy problem would become dissemination of this knowledge base to alter provider behaviour (and to focus future research work). Economists tend to focus on payment and price systems and the impact of these systems on provider and consumer behaviour. However, the knowledge base is limited, with what evidence there is favouring avoidance of fee-per-item payment systems and the use of capitation payments. The use of user charges (co-payments) to remedy provider inefficiencies in resource allocation is a tax on the sick and is much favoured by some strong provider groups (e.g., the pharmaceutical industry) as a means of weakening the global budget and maintaining their income.

The pharmaceutical industry is very effective in changing behaviour. The evidence that new treatments for depression (selective serotonin re-uptake inhibitors, or SSRIs) were no more efficacious and seemed to achieve no higher rates of patient compliance than the old treatments (tricyclics),[30] but were up to 20 times more expensive, had only transitory effects on share prices and rapid growth of the SSRI market. Thus evidence without dissemination and efficient incentives appears to have little chance of countervailing commercial marketing machines. There is an increased interest in dissemination and behaviour change, but deficiencies in knowledge about "what works" to change provider behaviour are striking.

Institutional Framework to Improve Efficiency

How can efficiency be improved, within a global budget and allocation based on ability to benefit? Two necessary but insufficient conditions for success are technology assessment and evaluation of alternative interventions to change behaviour, particularly the behaviour of physicians. Unfortunately, funds to create such knowledge bases are usually the first to be cut by governments, which generally fail to appreciate the fact that while the price of knowledge is high the cost of ignorance is greater!

Evidence about the design of alternative institutions that facilitate assessment of technology and application of the knowledge bases is also lacking. For economists, markets have intuitive appeal but the progression from theory to practice and its evaluation is in its very early stages. Such experimentation should always recognize that *markets are a means, not an end*. Without this recognition, market experiments may undermine equity and cost containment gains in many health care systems.

Overview

The paucity of information about market experiments in health care, and the willingness of many to ignore what evidence there is, continues to puzzle academic observers of the political marketplace. Such puzzlement is misplaced: most public policies are designed and implemented under conditions of great uncertainty and with little inclination to exploit the knowledge base. The primacy of the knowledge base for researchers, and their expectation that it should determine policy choice, is naïve for at least two reasons. Firstly, as Stigler (quoted in Fuchs) argued:

A scholar ought to be tolerably open minded, unemotional and rational. A reformer must promise paradise if his reform is adopted. Reform and research seldom march arm in arm.[31]

Secondly, public policy choices are informed by research evidence but determined by political expedience and social values. As Fuchs writes:

At the root of most of our major health problems are *value choices*. What kind of people are we? What kind of life do we want to lead? What kind of society do we want to build for our children and grandchildren? How much weight do we want to put on individual freedom? How much to equality? How much to material progress? How much to the realm of the spirit? How important is our own health to us? How important is our neighbour's health to us? The answers we give to these questions, as well as the guidance we get from economics, will and should shape health care policy.[32]

The dominance of US culture is such that reform proposals to deal with its inequity, inefficiency and cost inflation in health care are influencing policy choices elsewhere in the world. These countries have different perceptions of "the policy problem" (in particular, the primacy of the problem of inefficient resource allocation), having mitigated to varying degrees cost inflation and inequity. Yet they tend to adopt American policy changes precipitately and with little evaluation.

Market reforms have been implemented with great vigour and enthusiasm in the health care systems of many countries, and they have accompanied a greater appreciation of the need to identify and develop the knowledge base that is essential to informed policy choices. However, like previous "redisorganizations" of health care systems, the progress they induce in resource allocation seems slow and marginal. Cooper[33] described this in New Zealand as "jumping on the spot." The resources consumed by the internal market machine are large, but evidence about the gains they have produced is sparse. Decision makers attracted by the advocacy of "marketeers" should look before they leap and bear in mind always the advice of Mark Twain:

Whenever you are on the side of the majority, it is time to pause and reflect!

1. U. Reinhardt, "Tablemanners at the Health Care Feast," in D. Yaggy and W. A. Anylan (eds.), *Financing Health Care: Competition Versus Regulation* (Cambridge, Mass.: Ballinger, 1978); and "Comment on the Jackson Hole Initiatives for a Twenty-First Century American Health Care System," *Health Economics,* Vol. 2, no. 1 (1993), pp. 7–14.

2. A. Maynard and A. Williams, "Privatisation and the National Health Service," in J. Le Grand and R. Robinson (eds.), *Privatisation and the Welfare State* (London: George Allen & Unwin, 1984).

3. A. J. Culyer, A. Maynard and A. Williams, "Alternative Systems of Health Care Provision: An Essay on Motes and Beams," in M. Olson (ed.), *A New Approach to the Economics of Health Care* (Washington, DC: American Enterprise Institute for Public Policy Research, 1981), pp. 131–50.

4. A. Williams, "Need: An Economic Exegesis," in A. J. Culyer and K. Wright (eds.), *Economic Aspects of Health Services* (London: Martin Robertson, 1978).

5. See A. Cochrane, *Effectiveness and Efficiency* (London: Nuffield Provincial Hospitals Trust, 1972); and J. Bunker, J. Barnes and F. Mosteller, *Cost Risks and Benefits of Surgery* (New York: Oxford University Press, 1977).

6. J. E. Wennberg, "Future Directions for Small Area Variations," *Medical Care (Supplement),* Vol. 5, no. 31 (1993), pp. YS75–80.

7. S. J. Bernstein *et al.,* "The Appropriateness of the Use of Cardiovascular Procedures: British *Versus* US Perspectives," *International Journal of Technology Assessment in Health Care,* Vol. 9, no. 1 (1993), pp. 3–10.

8. R. H. Brook *et al.,* "Appropriateness of Acute Medical Care for the Elderly: An Analysis of the Literature," *Health Policy,* no. 14 (1990), pp. 225–42.

9. A. Smith, *An Inquiry into the Nature and Causes of the Wealth of Nations,* Vol. 1 (Oxford: Oxford University Press, 1776, 1976), p. 145.

10. See Smith, *An Inquiry into the Nature and Causes of the Wealth of Nations,* Vol. 1, p. 146.

11. R. H. Coase, *The Firm, the Market and the Law* (Chicago: University of Chicago Press, 1988), p. 10.

12. See A. C. Enthoven, *Health Plan: The Only Practical Solution to the Soaring Cost of Medical Care* (Reading, Mass.: Addison-Wesley, 1980); and *Reflections on the Management of the National Health Service* (London: Nuffield Provincial Hospitals Trust, 1985), Occasional Paper 5. See also P. M. Ellwood, A. C. Enthoven and L. Etheridge, "The Jackson Hole Initiatives for a Twenty-First Century American Health Care System," *Health Economics,* Vol. 1, no. 3 (1992), pp. 169–80.

13. See Ellwood, Enthoven and Etheridge, "The Jackson Hole Initiatives for a Twenty-First Century American Health Care System."

14. *Managed Competition II,* a proposal from the Jackson Hole Group (March 1994).

15. A. Maynard, "Competition in the UK National Health Service: Mission Impossible," *Health Policy,* no. 23 (1993), pp. 193–204; and A. Maynard, "Can Competition Enhance Efficiency in Health Care? Lessons from the Reform of the UK National Health Service," *Social Science and Medicine,* Vol. 39, no. 10 (1994), pp. 1433–45.

16. A. Maynard and A. Walker, "Managing the Medical Workforce: Time for Improvements?" *Health Policy* (forthcoming 1994).

17. Smith, *An Inquiry into the Nature and Causes of the Wealth of Nations,* Vol. 1, pp. 26–27.

18. A. Smith, *The Theory of Moral Sentiments* (Oxford: Oxford University Press, 1790, 1976), pp. 160–62.

19. A. Relman, "What Market Values Are Doing to Medicine," *The Atlantic,* Vol. 269, no. 3 (1992), pp. 98–106.

20. V. R. Fuchs, *The Future of Health Policy* (Cambridge, Mass.: Harvard University Press, 1993).

21. J. E. Thompson, "Fundamental Ethical Principles in Health Care," in C. Phillips (ed.), *Logic in Medicine* (London: Pitman, 1988).

22. Maynard, "Competition in the UK National Health Service."

23. R. Robinson and J. Le Grand (eds.), *Evaluating the NHS Reforms* (London: King's Fund Institute, 1994).

24. J. Lomas, "Teaching Old (and Not So Old) Docs New Tricks: Effective Ways to Implement Research Findings," CHEPA Working Paper Series no. 93–4, (Hamilton, Ont.: McMaster University, 1993).

25. D. G. Altman, "The Scandal for Poor Medical Research," *British Medical Journal,* Vol. 308 (1994), pp. 283–84.

26. P. C. Gotzsche, "Methodology and Overt and Hidden Bias in Reports of 196 Double Blind Trials of Nonsteroidal Anti-Inflammatory Drugs in Rheumatoid Arthritis," *Controlled Clinical Trials,* Vol. 10 (1989), pp. 31–56.

27. J. C. Bailar, "Bailar's Laws of Data Analysis," *Clinical Pharmacological and Therapeutics,* Vol. 20, no. 1 (1976), pp. 113–19.

28. N. Freemantle and A. Maynard, "Something Rotten in the State of Clinical and Economic Evaluations?" *Health Economics,* Vol. 3, no. 2 (March-April 1994), pp. 63–67.

29. J. Gabbay and A. Stevens, "Toward Investing in Health Gain," *British Medical Journal,* Vol. 308 (1994), pp. 1117–18.

30. F. Song *et al.,* "Selective Serotonin Re-Uptake Inhibitors: Meta-Analysis of Efficacy and Acceptability," *British Medical Journal,* Vol. 306 (1993), pp. 683–87. See also N. Freemantle *et al.,* "The Treatment of Depression in Primary Care," *Effective Health Care Bulletin* (Leeds: Leeds University School of Public Health, 1993).

31. V. Fuchs, "The Clinton Plan: A Researcher Examines Reform," *Health Affairs,* Vol. 13, no. 1 (Spring 1994), pp. 102–14.

32. V. Fuchs, *Who Shall Live?* (New York: Basic Books, 1974), p. 148.

33. M. H. Cooper, "Jumping on the Spot: Health Reform New Zealand Style," *Health Economics,* Vol. 3, no. 2 (March-April 1994), pp. 69–72.

Appendix

Idealized Health Care Systems

	Private	Public
Demand	1 Individuals are the best judges of their own welfare. 2 Priorities determined by own willingness and ability to pay. 3 Erratic and potentially catastrophic nature of demand mediated by private insurance. 4 Matters of equity to be dealt with elsewhere (e.g., in the tax and social security systems).	1 When ill, individuals are frequently imperfect judges of their own welfare. 2 Priorities determined by social judgements about need. 3 Erratic and potentially catastrophic nature of demand made irrelevant by provision of free services. 4 Since the distribution of income and wealth unlikely to be equitable in relation to the need for health care, the public health care system must be insulated from its influence.
Supply	1 Profit is the proper and effective way to motivate suppliers to respond to the needs of demanders. 2 Priorities determined by people's willingness and ability to pay and by the costs of meeting their wishes at the margin. 3 Suppliers have strong incentive to adopt least-cost methods of provision.	1 Professional ethics and dedication to public service are the appropriate motivation, focussing on success in curing or caring. 2 Priorities determined by where the greatest improvements in caring or curing can be effected at the margin. 3 Predetermined limit on available resources generates a strong incentive for suppliers to adopt least-cost methods of provision.
Adjustment mechanism	1 Many competing suppliers ensure that offer prices are kept low and reflect costs. 2 Well-informed consumers are able to seek out the most cost-effective form of treatment for themselves.	1 Central review of activities generates efficiency audit of service provision and management pressures keep the system cost-effective. 2 Well-informed clinicians are able to prescribe the most cost-effective form of treatment for each patient.

	3. If, at the price that clears the market, medical practice is profitable, more people will go into medicine, and hence supply will be demand-responsive.	3. If there is resulting pressure on some facilities or specialties, resources will be directed toward extending them.
	4. If, conversely, medical practice is unremunerative, people will leave it or stop entering it until the system returns to equilibrium.	4. Facilities or specialties on which pressure is slack will be slimmed down to release resources for other uses.
Success criteria	1. Consumers will judge the system by their ability to get someone to do what they demand, when, where and how they want.	1. Electorate judges the system by the extent to which it improves the health status of the population at large in relation to the resources allocated to it.
	2. Producers will judge the system by how good a living they can make out of it.	2. Producers judge the system by its ability to enable them to provide the treatments they believe to be cost-effective.

Appendix (continued)

Actual Health Care Systems

		Private	Public
Demand	1	Doctors act as agents, mediating demand on behalf of consumers.	Doctors act as agents, identifying need on behalf of patients.
	2	Priorities determined by the reimbursement rules of insurance funds.	Priorities determined by the doctor's own professional situation, by his assessment of the patient's condition and the expected trouble-making proclivities of the patient.
	3	Because private insurance coverage is itself a profit seeking activity, some risk rating is inevitable, hence coverage is incomplete and uneven, distorting personal willingness and ability to pay.	Freedom from direct financial contributions at the point of service, and absence of risk rating, enables patients to seek treatment for trivial or inappropriate conditions.
	4	Attempts to change the distribution of income and wealth independently are resisted as destroying incentives (one of which is the ability to buy better or more medical care if you are rich).	Attempts to correct inequities in the social and economic system by differential compensatory access to health services leads to recourse to health care in circumstances where it is unlikely to be a cost-effective solution to the problem.
Supply	1	What is most profitable to suppliers may not be what is most in the interests of consumers, and since neither consumers nor suppliers may be very clear about what is in the former's interests, this gives suppliers a range of discretion.	Personal professional dedication and public spirited motivation likely to be corroded and degenerate into cynicism if others, who do not share those feelings, are seen to be doing very well for themselves through blatantly self-seeking behaviour.
	2	Priorities determined by the extent to which consumers can be induced to part with their money, and by the costs of satisfying the pattern of "demand."	Priorities determined by what gives the greatest professional satisfaction.
	3	Profit motive generates a strong incentive toward market segmentation and price discrimination, and tie-in agreements with other professionals.	Since cost-effectiveness is not accepted as a proper medical responsibility, such pressures merely generate tension between the "professionals" and the "managers."

Adjustment mechanism	1 Professional ethical rules are used to make overt competition difficult.	1	Because it does not need elaborate cost data for billing purposes, it does not routinely generate much useful information on costs.
	2 Consumers denied information about quality and competence, and, since insured, may collude with doctors (against the insurance carriers) in inflating costs.	2	Clinicians know little about costs, and have no direct incentive to act on such information as they have, and sometimes even quite perverse incentives (i.e., cutting costs may make life more difficult or less rewarding for them).
	3 Entry into the profession made difficult and numbers restricted to maintain profitability.	3	Very little is known about the relative cost effectiveness of different treatments, and even where it is, doctors are wary of acting on such information until a general professional consensus emerges.
	4 If demand for service falls, doctors extend range of activities and push out neighbouring disciplines.	4	The phasing out of facilities which have become redundant is difficult because it often threatens the livelihood of some concentrated, specialized group and has identifiable people dependent on it, whereas the beneficiaries are dispersed and can only be identified as "statistics."
Success criteria	1 Consumers will judge the system by their ability to get someone to do what they need done without making them "medically indigent" and/or changing their risk rating too adversely.	1	Since the easiest aspect of health status to measure is life expectancy, the discussion is dominated by mortality data and mortality risks to the detriment of treatments concerned with non-life-threatening situations.
	2 Producers will judge the system by how good a living they can make out of it.	2	In the absence of accurate data on cost effectiveness, producers judge the system by the extent to which it enables them to carry out the treatments which they find the most exciting and satisfying.

SOURCE: A. Maynard and A. Williams, "Privatisation and the National Health Service," in J. Le Grand and R. Robinson (eds.), *Privatisation and the Welfare State* (London: George Allen & Unwin, 1984).

C L A S   R E H N B E R G

The Swedish Experience

with Internal Markets

Introduction

Health care has been one of the most rapidly expanding sectors in Sweden. From 1960 to 1982, expenditures rose continuously, from 4.7 to 9.1 percent of GDP. Employment in the health care field increased during the same period from 4.0 to 9.9 percent of total employment. An international comparison of health care costs during this period indicates similar trends in Canada and the United States. Table 1 shows the shares of health care expenditures and health care employment as a percentage of total employment for Sweden, Canada and the US.

Until the early 1980s, Sweden and the US devoted a larger share of their GDP to health care than did other countries, including Canada. Since the mid-1980s, this percentage has grown more rapidly in the US than in Sweden, but it has also risen in Canada. The difference between Swedish and US expenditures largely reflects differences in absolute and relative prices (wages). Sweden devotes a greater share of its employment to health care, and has more doctors per capita, but at the same time it devotes a significantly smaller share of its GDP to this sector.

Most of the expansion in Swedish health care had taken place in the public sector, represented by local county councils. Because of this

Table 1

Share of Health Care Expenditures in GDP, and Total Health Employment as a Percentage of Total Employment in Sweden, Canada and the US (1960-1990/91)

	Share of GDP				Share of Employment			
	1960	1970	1980	1991	1960	1970	1980	1990
Sweden	4.7	7.2	9.4	8.6	4.0	6.2	9.9	9.9
Canada	5.5	7.1	7.4	10.0	3.2	4.0	4.7	5.2
United States	5.3	7.4	9.2	13.4	2.7	3.7	5.3	6.3

NOTES: After 1985, expenditure for care of the mentally retarded was no longer included in the Swedish figures. This change in the definition of health care expenditure accounts for 0.6 percent of GDP. Final employment share figure for Canada is for 1985, not 1990.

SOURCE: OECD Health Data File.

decentralized structure, the central government had difficulty controlling costs. The county councils could at that time expand health care without considering the effects on the total economy. After 1985 the central government was able to enforce a small decrease in the share of Swedish GDP devoted to health care. Efforts to cope with this restraint on real resources led to a review of the efficiency, financing and organization of the system.

The Swedish health care system has historically relied on planning and coordination as a substitute for market mechanisms, a fundamental principle being that all citizens should have, as a matter of right, equal access to care regardless of where they live and their ability to pay. The structure of the system can to a large extent be explained by this history. The county councils were established in the 1960s, mainly to operate hospitals for somatic illnesses; the structure for outpatient care combined the services of private practitioners and district physicians paid by the State. Mental hospitals were managed and financed by the central government. During the last 25 years, several areas of responsibility have been transferred from the central government to the 23 county councils, the constituent populations of which vary from 60,000 to 1.6 million.

By the late 1980s, health care was dispensed chiefly from hospitals, primary health care centres and other facilities run by the county councils. Services contracted from external providers were very limited — mostly for highly specialized care obtained in another county. Contracting with external private providers has been very limited and foremost in ambulatory care. The system was a monolithic one, with all councils delivering care in a similar fashion. The county councils also have the power to levy a proportional income tax on their populations.

Health care, which is the sole responsibility of the county councils, accounts for 85 to 90 percent of a county's operating costs. Gradually, the counties have expanded the volume of their activities, and tasks have been transferred from the central government and the private sector. The county council has thus been transformed into a monopoly supplier of health care as well as a monopsonist. Private providers account for less than 10 percent of total delivery. Financing from the national Social Insurance System is used to pay for private health care. Private practitioners and dentists receive approximately 75 and 60 percent, respectively, of their revenues through the Social Insurance System. Private physicians account for 20 percent of all physician visits and private dentists for 50 percent of all dental treatments.

The general health of the population is excellent: life expectancy and infant and prenatal mortality rates place Sweden among the healthiest countries in the world. However, it should be noted that these positive vital statistics cannot be attributed solely to the health care *system*. Regarding subtler measures, such as quality of the health care *process* and outcomes, attention paid to *consumer preferences,* etc., the picture is less clear. At any rate, public opinion polls show that Swedes have a high regard for their health care system.

Providers in the public system have been granted a monopoly position so that they can take advantage of large-scale production and avoid wasteful duplication, and because such a structure is consistent with the requirements of the planning model. Public providers have not been subject to much competition: the county councils have contracted outside the public sector for health services only to a limited extent. The debate of the 1980s pointed to integration problems as well as decreased efficiency. Several studies showed productivity differentials between public and private providers, to the disadvantage of the former.[1] Part of this difference was attributed to a greater use of non-physician labour with no change in the use of physician labour — yet with similar levels of service. In addition, significant differences in productivity were found *within* the public sector.[2] The absence of competition has been interpreted as an important contributor to these results. The present health care reforms in Sweden must be seen against this background.

Until the late 1980s, the budget process contained costs by determining the allocation of resources based on past use of input factors (labour, equipment, supplies, etc.). By closely controlling the use of these resources the system became successful in terms of cost containment. This approach, however, provided little information with which to improve efficiency, and gave management incentives to spend their entire budgets.[3] Furthermore, resources were distributed across geographical areas in a manner that was poorly related to needs, perhaps in response to the interests of existing providers. Changes in medical practice were not always followed by a corresponding reallocation of resources. The absence of management information systems and incentives for cost effectiveness might explain the inability to redistribute resources. The maldistribution and inefficiencies could have contributed to deficiencies such as long waiting lists for surgical procedures in many locations.

Lack of consumer choice became a political issue as well. In 1985, the Government Committee on Power and Democracy in Sweden showed, based on 2,000 interviews, that education, health care and child day care received low scores regarding ability to influence service and to choose provider.[4] The study also showed that citizens considered the actual quality of care satisfactory. But, combined with problems such as waiting lists and the need to cope with stagnant economic growth, the study helped precipitate discussions on the efficiency of the system that resulted in a series of reform proposals. Abolition of the county councils has been proposed, as well as a transfer of responsibility for health care financing to either the municipalities or the Social Insurance System.

REFORM OF THE SWEDISH HEALTH CARE SYSTEM

In the 1990s, a large deficit and negative economic growth for three years, combined with a change in political orientation, heightened interest in finding new ways of structuring and financing health care. Concerns about both consumer choice and efficiency in the provision of health services made it necessary to change the role of the county politicians, who as *de facto* owners of the local systems too often represented provider (especially medical profession) interests rather than those of the citizen-consumers.

Several county councils responded to these and other concerns by making structural changes. A common principle in the reforms has been to make politicians concentrate on the interests of citizens by separating the consumer/purchaser and provider roles within the county councils. The providers in these counties remain under public ownership, but politicians have decided not to be represented on the boards of hospitals and health centres. They therefore have less decision-making power at the operational level.

The movement toward market mechanisms in public health care can be summarized as encompassing the following features:
- Collective purchasing units
- Consumer freedom of choice
- Provider competition
- Contracts and performance-based reimbursement
- Provider autonomy

At one time, changes to the organizational and financial structure of county councils were determined centrally. During the 1960s and 1970s, even management control systems were designed and implemented by the Federation of County Councils. Now those systems, and basic governing structures, are being designed at the county level and Swedish versions of the internal market consequently show greater variety.

As late as 1993 only six of the 24 county councils had implemented models featuring a purchaser-provider split. In 1994, more than half of the counties still rely on the traditional budget process for allocating resources. Some, however, have adopted forms of decentralization and formula budgeting instead. They have created collective purchasing units funded according to population characteristics (number of inhabitants, age, etc.). These units purchase health services from the county's providers, but can purchase from external providers not connected to the county council as well.[5]

Thus Dalarna and Bohuslän decentralized the purchasing function to primary health districts ranging in population from 6,000 to 50,000. Stockholm instead established large districts within the county council, to act on behalf of the county councils and indirectly the consumers. Sörmland and Östergötland did not create new regions, but established central purchasing agencies. Table 2 shows some characteristics of these county councils.

Purchasing agencies, then, may be buying services on new terms, through performance-related reimbursements such as fee-for-service or fee-per-diagnosis. Such arrangements have been adopted slowly and applied where most appropriate. Table 3 shows that this form of purchaser-provider split was first applied to surgical specialties. Specialties with a higher degree of uncertainty about costs and outcome and in which the output is difficult to observe (psychiatry, geriatrics) are being included more slowly.

In addition to these county-level reforms, the national government introduced the Family Doctor Reform,[6] under which every citizen is granted the right to enrol with one family doctor. In the Swedish context this was presented as an expansion of choice. Previously, primary care had been administered by staffed public health centres, which paid a salary to their own staff. Individuals were assigned to the health centre responsible for their catchment area. In the larger cities they could use the services of remaining private practitioners under the terms of contracts with the county councils. These practitioners are now also entitled

Table 2

Population and Size
of Some Swedish County Councils

County Councils That Have Introduced Internal Markets	Population	As Percentage of National Population	Km^2	As Percentage of National Total
Dalarna	290 245	3.3	28 193.6	6.9
Stockholm	1 669 840	19.2	6 487.6	1.6
Örebro	274 325	3.2	8 518.6	2.1
Östergötland	408 268	4.7	10 562.0	2.6
Bohuslän	314 038	3.6	5 140.7	1.3
Sörmland	257 858	3.0	6 060.4	1.5
Total in Country	8 692 013		410 930	

Table 3

Adoption of Internal Markets
by County Councils in Sweden

Year	County Council	Specialty
1991	Dalarna Stockholm	Somatic hospital care Surgery, two hospitals
1992	Dalarna Stockholm Örebro Östergötland	Psychiatry Some surgery Some surgery Dental care
1993	Stockholm Bohuslän Östergötland Örebro Sörmland	All surgery/medicine All health care All health care Somatic hospital care All health care

to enter the system of family doctors and compete with public physicians. The Family Doctor Reform in essence lets a person choose a doctor within the health centres as well, but patients must pay extra if they see a different doctor. In practice, county councils have allowed a patient to switch doctors at any time.

Under these new arrangements, physicians are allowed to keep out-of-pocket fees, which are expected to contribute between 20 and 30 percent of their income. Physicians will also receive capitation payments, adjusted for age, for each patient on their lists. Prescribed medicines are reimbursed separately by the central government.

It must be noted that these reforms do not change the way in which health care is financed. The principles of fairness and equity are strongly ingrained in Swedish health care policy, which considers it essential that factors such as age, sex, income or place of residence do not become the basis for discrimination. There is general agreement that financing of health care should be based on ability to pay, regardless of individual risk. Direct consumer charges are nominal (CDN$17–$34) per physician visit. Fees are still regulated by the central government, which stipulates a maximum (CDN$43). This gives the county councils some latitude in using fees as a rationing instrument. There is also an annual ceiling of CDN$280. Consumer out-of-pocket expenses account for 10 percent of total health care expenditures (including drugs, dental care, etc.).

REGULATION AND COMPETITION AMONG PROVIDERS

A major reason for separating the financial and provider functions is to introduce competition among providers, since an important objective of the reforms is to break up the monopoly held by public providers. The market solutions being implemented do not involve the introduction of "pure" markets; rather, they create a kind of internal market or "quasi market," whereby tax financing of health care is retained but a form of managed competition is introduced into the system.

Market Structure

For the market allocation of a service to be efficient, the market concerned must be competitive. A number of conditions must then be met: there must be many providers and purchasers, it must be possible to freely enter and exit the market, and so on.

The market structure within the county councils differs in several respects from a conventional competitive one. Providers are given considerable freedom to organize the delivery of health care. This autonomy is, however, circumvented by regulations regarding public ownership. For example, a decision to close down a hospital or primary health centre must be sanctioned by county politicians, and large investments in facilities and equipment are controlled by regional political boards. Decisions about "pure" production issues, such as the mix of labour and other inputs and investments below a certain limit, have been decentralized to local managers. Still, in practice, politicians have not followed the recommendations of hospital managers to lay off public employees during periods of recession. The shift toward competition is a process in which the rules concerning provider autonomy are perceived by many production managers to be changeable and arbitrary. Nevertheless, providers have become considerably more autonomous and less subject to detailed regulation. A more professional leadership, under which managers are recruited from the private sector, serves to strengthen this process. Hospitals and other institutions are reimbursed through contracts or agreements with purchasing units. This process can be described as competitive tendering, with mainly public providers competing among themselves.

In those counties, such as Dalarna, that have decentralized purchasing substantially, the local purchasing unit cooperates closely with the primary physicians in its area to purchase hospital and specialist services. The provision of primary care is thus integrated with the work of the purchasing unit. This requires a tradeoff between primary and specialist services at the local level. Hospitals tend to serve larger areas, so each is seeking business from several purchasers. But there remain risks of a provider monopoly. Where counties have created central purchasing agencies, their monopsony power has been justified as necessary to counter the power of large providers such as hospitals. However, this also gives the purchasers a pure monopoly position regarding local providers such as primary care physicians.

Table 4 summarizes the range of economic relationships. Clearly the requirements for a competitive market are far from being met. Still, the examples of reforms are a departure from a system based on administrative coordination; for instance, the negotiation process itself has raised issues of quality that had not been explicitly considered

Table 4
The Purchaser/Provider Relationship

PROVIDERS / PURCHASERS	Hospitals	Primary Health Care
Local Units	Monopoly Providers	Vertical Integration
Central Units	Bilateral Monopoly	Monopsony Purchasers

under the previous budget process.

Competition among providers may refer to price as well as quality. Experience so far shows that prices are fixed administratively and decided upon centrally by the county councils. Negotiation in a marketplace involving several purchasers and providers has not been tested, even in subsectors characterized by a system of multiple providers and purchasers, such as primary health care. Overall, competition has focussed on accessibility and quality of the service provided. This form of non-price competition has created the incentive for providers to become more sensitive to customer satisfaction. Not surprisingly, the incentives to treat patients have in some subsectors caused an increase in total utilization of care, and thus costs. To counter this effect, competition has been accompanied by various budget restrictions. Some contracts between purchasers and providers specify a ceiling on utilization of health services.

Private Providers and Entry to the Market

The introduction of competition among *public* providers has also opened up the market to new *private* providers. Several of the county councils implementing internal markets have given private providers the opportunity to tender for contracts, although in practice these usually go to the incumbents. Large investments and uncertainty about the competitive neutrality of the public purchasers have made investors cautious about entering the market, especially in the hospital sector. The Family Doctor Reform also allows private practitioners to enrol patients, removing the barriers to the primary care market for new providers. In this market a large investment is not required, hence entry is less costly than in the hospital sector. Still, efficiency also requires that it be possible to exit the market — i.e., providers should be exposed to the risk of bankruptcy. A major problem of the Family Doctor Reform for the county councils concerns publicly employed primary care physicians who do not enrol enough patients. Their status as employees implies that they cannot be laid off even if they fail to meet the enrolment quota. This controversial issue led to a physician strike in the spring of 1994. The Federation of County Councils and the Swedish Medical Association still disagree on how to handle publicly employed physicians who fail to enrol enough patients. Hence the county councils are faced with a situation of free entry for private practitioners but no exit for publicly employed family doctors. New forms of public physician associations may therefore be required.

It is too early to determine the extent to which the introduction of competition and performance-related reimbursement has changed provider behaviour. Previously, public providers referred to long waiting lists to gain access to increased budget resources, even though official waiting lists did not always correspond with the actual number of individuals waiting for treatment. This process has disappeared.[7] Under a reimbursement system based on performance, providers must now increase their workload to attract more resources. An increase in productivity has been observed in some counties. The Stockholm county council also reports a greater increase in hospital admissions and faster reduction and turnover of acute-care beds when compared to those county councils that still rely on the budget process.[8] Also, several case studies show a drop in use of hospital ancillary services and greater staff awareness concerning the financial situation of their provider unit. Interview studies indicate that physicians pay more attention to costs.[9] From the consumer perspective, improved service and accessibility have been reported. No results have been reported concerning quality indicators. However, the general opinion is that while there has been increased *interest* in quality of care, there have not been any significant changes in quality due to introduction of the internal market.

CONTRACTUAL RELATIONSHIPS AND INFORMATION

Interaction between the consumer and provider sides within the county councils takes place in an internal market (or quasi market). In this internal market the supply side comprises public institutions with a certain degree of autonomy over operations. In addition, private providers compete for public contracts in some specialties. The demand side comprises two actors: purchasing units and individual consumers. The purchasing unit acts as agent for the consumer and signs the contracts on the demand side. Individual consumers influence resource allocation through their choice of providers. Hence, the providers compete for two kinds of customers.

Purchasing units receive their revenues on a capitation basis. They sign service contracts with public and private providers. The intent is for purchasing units to maximize the health status of their client population within the limitations of their budget. It is difficult to judge the extent to which this objective is being met, or whether the purchasers tend to pursue their own agendas: as monopoly purchasers they have no clear incentives to act in the interests of the citizen; still, the interests of the citizen are central to the political mandate. The change in the role of the politician — from acting in the interests of both consumer and provider to acting as pure purchasing agent for the citizen — might lead to an increased focus on the interests of the consumer.

Bilateral Monopoly and Lock-in Effects

In the past, the county councils built hospitals, nursing homes and primary care centres within a defined catchment area. The fact that the location of facilities implied a monopoly position for several providers is now hampering the creation of a competitive environment. The problem of dominant providers is greatest in the hospital sector, since all cities except the three largest ones have only one hospital. Furthermore, considering that Sweden is a sparsely populated country it is not clear that a competitive market with a greater number of providers would be more allocatively efficient, since the advantages of large-scale production probably exist in the hospital sector. However, a solution could be found by increasing the use of distant providers and/or by exposing incumbent providers to competition. Several polls have shown that citizens are reluctant to travel distances of 20 or 30 kilometres for health care. In regions where several county councils agree on free choice of providers across boundaries, however, there have been changes in patient behaviour. In the case of natural monopolies, the purchasers can use the potential for competition — that is, the opportunity for providers to enter the market relatively cost-free ("contestable market").[10] Nonetheless, such an arrangement involves investment problems as well as uncertainty among potential providers about the neutrality of public purchasers when choosing between public and private providers.

Access to information also affects the efficiency of internal markets. A condition for a market relationship is that both purchaser and provider have accurate information about costs, prices, quality, etc. Given a more autonomous position, competing providers would be reluctant to share all information about costs and required resources. Providers might engage in what Williamson[11] calls "opportunistic behaviour" — i.e., one party realizes gains by concealing information and thereby imposing costs on the other party. There are examples, on both the purchasing and provision sides, of previously public information becoming confidential.

In general, providers have better access to information than do purchasers. Management control systems are naturally controlled by the providers. Also, the more experienced managers have been recruited to run larger units such as hospitals. Thus at the initial stage, when market mechanisms are introduced, providers are much better prepared to negotiate and bargain. When the separate purchasing units are established, accounting and management staff are recruited, as well as specialists in epidemiology and social medicine. Informational asymmetry may diminish over time, and purchasers in some county councils claim they are in a better position to bargain with providers now than they were under the previous budget system.

Contract Structure

The traditional allocation of resources via the budget process is being replaced by a system of contractual relationships between purchasers and providers. The nature and level of the service, as well as the method of reimbursement, are specified in the contracts. The contracts fall into two main categories:

1. In the block contract, the purchaser pays a yearly sum in return for access to a defined range of services. The capacity of a specific service is defined in this type of contract, which is found primarily in those medical specialties in which output is difficult to verify (psychiatry, geriatrics). One problem with this type of arrangement is that the contract is incomplete, which leaves the door open to opportunism. With major information asymmetry in these specialties, both provider and purchaser are placed at risk, although the purchaser faces greater risk. The purchaser has limited opportunity to monitor output and outcome of services, while the provider risks unexpected cost increases due to uncertain utilization patterns. An important feature of these contracts is performance targets, such as waiting lists that entitle the patient to treatment within a specified period of time. This type of performance target was initiated by the central government and the Federation of County Councils in 1992 for a set of surgical procedures. The councils have continued to include it in their contracts, and it has been judged to have significant influence over provider behaviour. The earlier waiting times, sometimes years, mainly for surgical procedures, have been eliminated or reduced to

months. During 1992, waiting lists for surgical procedures were reduced by 27 percent.[12]

2. The performance-related contract is used mainly in surgical specialties and internal medicine, where output can be observed and forms the basis for reimbursement. Some county councils use the Diagnosis Related Group (DRG) classification, whereas others use measures such as admissions and visits. Additional resources are allocated separately for units that treat difficult cases of above-average severity and/or have education or research commitments. These contracts are sometimes combined with a ceiling for total care that is intended to control costs. Prices are generally based on average costs, but pricing based on marginal costs is used above a certain level of activity. The drawbacks of performance-related contracts include price uncertainty (as no market price exists) and the incentive to over-use.

Administrative Costs

A central issue in contractual relationships is the volume of administrative activity. Administrative costs accompany both integrated systems and contract relationships between independent buyers and sellers. It should also be noted that to focus exclusively on lowering the level of administrative costs can generate problems in controlling utilization and thus total costs. For example, the Swedish Social Insurance System costs little to run but has difficulty controlling use by private practitioners. Generally, insurance systems with individual enrolment and individual premiums have higher administrative costs (table 5).

Table 5 shows that monopoly insurers enjoy lower administrative costs. The share of spending devoted to administrative costs has not increased substantially with the introduction of internal markets. Since the present reforms do not alter universal coverage and do not include individual enrolment with individual risk evaluation, it is unlikely that these costs will increase drastically. However, experience suggests that *ex ante* administrative costs — those that precede production — are greater in agreements with external providers. On the other hand, *ex post* costs — control and evaluation costs — are greater in integrated systems. County councils with multiple purchasing units fear the expansion of administrative activities. Those costs could be reduced by introducing cooperation among small local units.

In all county councils with a purchaser-provider split, patients have

Table 5

Administrative Costs as a Share of Total Expenditures for Different Third-Party Payers

Health Care System	Share of Total Expenditures
Sweden	
County Councils	
Stockholm	4.0%
Dalarna	3.0%
Social Insurance System	1.5%
(private physicians)	
United States	
Medicare	2.1%
Medicaid	3.2-11.8%
HMO	2.5-7.0%
Private Insurance	
Business	5.5-40%
Individual	40%

SOURCES: K.E. Thorpe, "Inside the Black Box of Administrative Costs," *Health Affairs*, Vol. 11 (Summer 1992), pp. 41-55; and C. Rehnberg, "Administrationskostnader inom hälso-och Sjukvården," in SOU, *Hälso-och sjukvarden i fram tiden-Tre modeller* (Stockholm: Social Department, 1993).

been given a high degree of freedom to choose providers. Hence there is a coordination problem on the demand side. Providers must deal not only with formal contracts signed by an agent on behalf of citizens, but, at the same time, with individual choices. These two signals are not always concurrent. Individuals may choose different providers or consume a higher volume of health services than specified in the contract. No strategy has yet been able to deal adequately with the different signals sent to providers.

FREEDOM OF CHOICE AND CONSUMER SOVEREIGNTY

Swedish health services have been deficient with regard to consumer choice. Organization of health care based on geographic catchment area and population-based responsibility limited opportunities for patients to influence their personal situations. Unlike patients in many other countries, Swedish patients could visit a hospital clinic without a referral from their primary care physician, but they had little say in the choice of physician or clinic. Several inquiries identified patient dissatisfaction in this area.

Freedom of choice can refer to choice of insurer and/or choice of provider for a specific illness. Changes of the former type have not been seriously discussed in Sweden. The equity principle, the problem of preferred risk selection, and high transaction costs in systems with individual enrolment have been used as arguments for a universal insurance contract.[13] Consequently, all citizens are taxed by the county in which they live and cannot opt out of the system.

The new reforms have substantially increased the individual's ability to choose provider. Two alternatives have been considered regarding how this choice can be arranged. The first is to design the system of reimbursement so that the money directly follows the patient. Such a voucher-type arrangement would force providers to profile themselves in order to attract patients. The second alternative is to use patient choice as a "guidance" system in the negotiations between providers and purchasing units. Resources would continue to be allocated to health services following collective decisions, but by virtue of their choice of provider patients would be making their preferences known.

The Family Doctor Reform gives the patient the right to choose primary care provider. This increased choice is also central to several of the internal market models introduced by the county councils. Several councils allow the patient to choose among public and private providers (physicians as well as hospital clinics). The choice is not completely free, however, but is limited by the contracts signed by purchasing units. Agreements have been signed between some county councils allowing patients to obtain care across boundaries. One such example is the cooperation among county councils in Western Sweden, the effects of which are shown in table 6.

The net number of bed-days constitutes one to 10 percent of the total number of bed-days produced in the county councils of Western Sweden. Overall, patient choice of provider, which is limited in supply, as specified in contracts with purchasing units, has been the most powerful means of changing provider behaviour. Many councils report significant improvement in accessibility and service. However, this has limited effect on total resource allocation. Some two to five percent of total resources are reportedly redistributed due to consumer choice. Still, this probably under-estimates consumer impact on provider behaviour. With a voucher-type arrangement, whereby patient choice influences resource allocation, providers face a risk of losing patients and revenues. This effect cannot be observed directly by changes in patient flow.

The equity principle has been a major argument for retaining public financing of health care. In that respect, the introduction of internal markets does not affect accessibility. Universal insurance coverage and low patient fees serve to guarantee equal access. It has been argued, however, that the equity principle could be violated in an internal market. Since purchasing units would be pressured to use resources as efficiently as possible, they would concentrate on acute care, where treatment outcomes are observable. This could occur at the expense of chronic psychiatric and geriatric care, and deficiencies in the reimbursement system for severe cases could reinforce such discrimination. However, there are no studies indicating changes to this effect in resource allocation.

CONCLUSION

Implementation of internal markets in public health care is at such an early stage that it is impossible to determine the long-term consequences in terms of efficiency and equity. The experience so far can tell us about the structure of the internal market and describe the process of

Table 6

Net Result of Cross-Boundary Flow of Patients in the Western Region, Short-Term Acute Care (Bed-Days)

County Council	1991	1992	1993
Halland	-14,920	-17,337	-16,102
Bohus	+28,102	+30,062	+26,294
Älvsborg	-32,291	-35,456	-34,647
Skaraborg	-1,389	-1,684	-4,516
Göteborg	+20,498	+24,415	+28,981
Total Bed-Days	116,911	136,670	146,234
Annual Change		(+17%)	(+7%)

SOURCE: Planeringsnämnden i Västsverige, *Data över Patientstrommar* (Stockholm 1993)

implementation. It has been introduced successively, beginning in surgery and those subsectors characterized by observable outputs and a low degree of uncertainty. Even if the models are designed to encourage competition and purchaser units are allowed to buy from external providers, most services are provided by hospitals and other production units owned by county councils. Private providers have been reluctant to enter the market, probably because they are uncertain about the competitive neutrality of the purchasers.

In the discussion of market-oriented reforms a number of concepts have been used to analyze the market structure. As we have seen, the internal market in health care differs in several respects from a conventional competitive market. In figure 1 these concepts are used to summarize the change from a traditional planning model to one of internal markets in Swedish health care.

As shown in figure 1, several characteristics found in a competitive market do not exist in the internal market model. The shift toward market mechanisms concerns mainly the use of financial incentives through new ways of reimbursing providers. Still, prices are centrally regulated and controlled in most county councils. The second important change is the increased freedom for the consumer to choose provider. This voucher-type arrangement is reported to have a great effect on provider behaviour. The stipulation in contracts regarding maximum waiting times for specific procedures also strengthens the position of the consumer. Accessibility has been improved and waiting lists have been reduced in size.

Regarding the competitiveness of the market, several regulatory mechanisms are still in place. The mechanisms for entering and exiting the market are not developed. In general, the market structure can be described as regulated competition among public providers.

The market-oriented reforms in health care have affected the principles of resource allocation in this sector. Studies are nonetheless needed in order to identify which mechanisms contribute to increased efficiency and changes in patterns of utilization. The shorter waiting lists, etc., are interpreted as relating to the introduction of internal markets. On the other hand, similar trends are reported from county councils that rely on the traditional models; however, this could be considered a spillover effect, since providers in those county councils are aware of the shift toward the market model.

Figure 1
The Planning and Quasi-Market Models

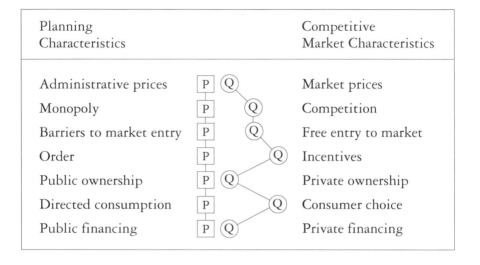

Planning Characteristics		Competitive Market Characteristics
Administrative prices	P Q	Market prices
Monopoly	P Q	Competition
Barriers to market entry	P Q	Free entry to market
Order	P Q	Incentives
Public ownership	P Q	Private ownership
Directed consumption	P Q	Consumer choice
Public financing	P Q	Private financing

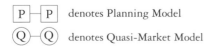

P—P   denotes Planning Model

Q—Q   denotes Quasi-Market Model

As in any market, regulations and other arrangements between the consumers and producers of health care are part of the learning process for each party. The efficiency gains made in the internal markets will depend on the nature of the market that will evolve. Finally, the problems with internal markets must be weighed against those encountered with the previous model, which was itself far from perfect.[14]

1. B. Jönsson, T. Faresjö and I. Westerberg, "Produktivitet i privat och offentlig tandvård" [Productivity in private and public dental care], *DsFi* (Stockholm), no. 27 (1983); and "Jämförande studie av privat och offentlig vård" [Comparison of private and public health care], *Landstingsförbundet* (Stockholm, 1985).

2. B. Lindgren and P. Roos, "Produktions- kostnads-och produktivitet-sutveckling inom affentligt bedriven hälso- och sjukvård 1960-1989" [The development of production, costs, and productivity in public health care], *DsFi* (Stockholm), no. 3 (1983).

3. B. Jönsson and C. Rehnberg, *Effektivare sjukvård* [More efficient medical care] (Stockholm: Norstedts, 1987).

4. O. Petersson, A. Westholm and G. Blomberg, *Medborgarnas makt* [The power of the citizens] (Stockholm: Carlsson Bokförlag, 1987).

5. The model of a purchaser-provider split shares several features with the National Health Service reform in the United Kingdom. In Sweden, however, the hospitals, which are owned by the county councils, have less autonomy than do the British hospital trusts.

6. This reform is similar to the British GP fundholding system.

7. "Jämförelstal för landstingen 1992" [Comparative statistics for the county councils in 1992], *Landstingsförbundet* (Stockholm, 1993).

8. E. Forsberg and J. Calltorp, "Ekonomiska incitament förändrar sjukvården" [Economic incentives imply changes in health care], *Läkartidningen,* Vol. 90 (1993), pp. 2611–14.

9. E. Jonsson, "Har den s.k. Stockholmsmodellen genererat mer vard for pengarna? — En jämforande utvärdering" [Does the Stockholm model generate more services for money? — A comparative evaluation], 1994 mimeo.

10. See W. J. Baumol, J. G. Panzar and R. D. Willig, *Contestable Markets and the Theory of Industry Structure* (New York: Harcourt Brace Jovanovich, 1982).

11. O. E. Williamson, *The Economic Institutions of Capitalism* (New York: Free Press, 1985).

12. "Jämförelstal för landstingen 1992."
13. The Dutch example shows that this can be accomplished even if there is competition among insurance plans.
14. This research was supported by grants from the Federation of County Councils.

R I C H A R D   B .   S A L T M A N

THE ROLE OF COMPETITIVE INCENTIVES

IN RECENT REFORMS OF

NORTHERN EUROPEAN HEALTH SYSTEMS

INTRODUCTION

Health care systems in Northern European countries (defined here as the Nordic Countries plus the United Kingdom) are widely acknowledged to be among the most successful in the industrialized world. These systems have consistently contributed to high (Nordic Countries) or relatively high (UK) international rankings on infant mortality and longevity indexes, and continue to command high levels of support among their populations.

Northern European systems have achieved these results with a relatively modest commitment of financial resources. As indicated in table 1, health expenditures in the UK, Norway, Denmark and Finland[1] were at or below the OECD average, while Sweden's expenditures fell during the 1980–91 period.

Despite broad success on expenditure and outcome indexes, Northern European countries, like most OECD member States, are engaged in a substantial re-examination of the structure and the organization of their health services. Major structural changes have been under way in the UK, Finland and Sweden for several years, while Denmark has hesitantly begun a process of change that will likely evolve into a

Table 1

Total Health Expenditures as a Percentage of Gross Domestic Product (GDP), 1985-91

	1985	1986	1987	1988	1989	1990	1991	Compound Annual Rate of Growth
Australia	7.7%	8.0%	7.8%	7.7%	7.8%	8.2%	8.6%	1.9%
Austria	8.1	8.3	8.4	8.4	8.4	8.3	8.4	0.6
Belgium	7.4	7.6	7.7	7.7	7.6	7.6	7.9	1.1
Canada	8.5	8.8	8.9	8.8	9.0	9.5	10.0	2.7
Denmark	6.3	6.0	6.3	6.5	6.5	6.3	6.5	0.5
Finland	7.2	7.4	7.4	7.2	7.2	7.8	8.9	3.6
France	8.5	8.5	8.5	8.6	8.7	8.8	9.1	1.1
Germany	8.7	8.6	8.7	8.8	8.3	8.3	8.5	-0.4
Greece	4.9	5.4	5.2	5.0	5.4	5.4	5.2	1.0
Iceland	7.1	7.8	8.0	8.6	8.6	8.3	8.4	2.8
Ireland	8.2	8.1	7.7	7.3	6.9	7.0	7.3	-1.9
Italy	7.0	6.9	7.4	7.6	7.6	8.1	8.3	2.9

Japan	6.5	6.6	6.7	6.6	6.6	6.7	6.8	0.8
Luxembourg	6.8	6.7	7.3	7.2	6.9	7.2	7.2	1.0
Netherlands	8.0	8.1	8.3	8.2	8.1	8.2	8.3	0.6
New Zealand	6.5	6.7	7.0	7.1	7.2	7.3	7.6	2.6
Norway	6.4	7.1	7.4	7.7	7.4	7.4	7.6	2.9
Portugal	7.0	6.6	6.8	7.1	7.2	6.7	6.8	-0.5
Spain	5.7	5.6	5.7	6.0	6.3	6.6	6.7	2.7
Sweden	8.8	8.5	8.6	8.6	8.6	8.6	8.6	-0.4
Switzerland	7.6	7.6	7.7	7.8	7.5	7.8	7.9	0.6
Turkey	2.8	3.5	3.6	3.8	3.9	4.0	4.0	6.1
United Kingdom	6.0	6.1	6.1	6.1	6.1	6.2	6.6	1.6
United States	10.5	10.7	10.9	11.1	11.5	12.2	13.2	3.9
OECD average	7.2%	7.3%	7.4%	7.5%	7.5%	7.6%	7.9%	1.6%

SOURCES: OECD *Health Systems: Facts and Trends* (Paris: Organisation for Economic Co-operation and Development, 1993); and S. Letsch *et al.*, "National Health Expenditures, 1991," *Health Care Financing Review* (Winter 1992).

Taken from G.J. Schieber, J.-P. Poullier and L.M. Greenwald, "Health Spending, Delivery, and Outcomes in OECD Countries," *Health Affairs*, Vol. 12, no. 2 (Summer 1993), p. 121.

NOTES: Health Canada uses a slightly different definition of gross domestic product (GDP) from that used in GDP figures reported to the OECD. Using the Health Canada GDP figures produces slightly different health-to-GDP ratios; these alternative ratios are 8.5 percent for 1985, 8.8 percent for 1986, 8.8 percent for 1987, 8.7 percent for 1988, 8.9 percent for 1989, 9.4 percent for 1990 and 9.9 percent for 1991.

major reconfiguration as well.

Analytically speaking, these changes are not generally taking place on the *finance* side of health care systems. No Northern European country has introduced competitive or market-style incentives into the tax-based mechanisms they have historically used to raise health sector revenues. This remains true even in the UK, despite Margaret Thatcher's intention to introduce competitive private insurance during her 1987–88 Cabinet review of the National Health Service (NHS).[2] Rather, the UK, Finland and Sweden, and to a lesser degree Denmark, are introducing specific market mechanisms in pursuit of micro-efficiencies on the *production* side of their health systems, and in the *allocation mechanisms* that distribute revenue to the producing institutions.[3] This pattern is broadly consistent with the approach to health care reform in most OECD countries, with the notable exceptions of the Clinton Administration proposal in the United States and the discontinued Simons Plan in the Netherlands.

This paper will explore the role of competitive incentives in recent reform initiatives in Northern European countries. After a brief overview of the finance side of these systems, the paper will concentrate on changes made in the production of health services and in the allocation mechanisms that connect finance and production. Emphasis will be placed on the UK, Finland and Sweden, which are in the midst of the most extensive changes.

REFORMS ON THE FINANCE SIDE

Northern European systems have traditionally been financed from one or more public sector tax bases. The British NHS, as an arm of the government, is fully financed nationally from general tax revenues. There are no co-payments for general practitioner (GP) or inpatient hospital services. Despite recent discussions about the sale of hospital land on the commercial market as well as service contracts with private insurers, the only realistic sources of additional funds are patient co-payments for eyeglasses and certain outpatient prescription drugs (for patients of working age with non-chronic conditions). While the NHS has some pay-beds, independent analysts have argued that these lose rather than make money.[4]

The Nordic pattern is that 50–70 percent of health revenues are obtained from personal income taxes levied by the government that owns and operates the provider institutions (regional government in Norway, Sweden and Denmark, municipal in Finland). The remaining funds come mostly from general revenues raised nationally through the value-added tax (VAT), tariffs on imported goods and personal and corporate income taxes. These national funds typically are distributed to regional and local governments through one or more block grants, at least a portion of which is intended to compensate for inequities in regional or local tax bases. There may be other national grants as well: in Sweden, for example, there are payments for medical education and training, payments from the national sickness insurance fund for outpatient physician visits and payments from municipal to regional governments to cover "finished" elderly patients not yet accepted into local home care (see below).

In the Nordic Countries, a small percentage of revenue comes from patient co-payments. In Sweden, the total amount of these co-payments has been restricted by national legislation to 1,600 SEK (about US $200 or CDN $280) per individual per year, and in recent years has come to about two percent of total county health-related revenues.[5] In Finland, there were no co-payments for primary care or hospital services until 1993, when difficult economic circumstances led the conservative government to introduce two types of relatively small, service-related co-payments.[6]

None of these countries is planning to introduce competitive incentives on the *finance* side of their health care systems. On the contrary: all are keeping their single-source payer systems, whether national (UK), regional (Sweden, Denmark) or municipal (Finland). What few changes are occurring are broadly regulatory in nature, involving re-alignment of responsibilities among the various levels of authority.

The only recent financing change of note was the ÄDEL reform introduced in Sweden in January 1992, in which financial as well as operating responsibility for residential care for the elderly was transferred from Sweden's 26 counties to its 284 municipalities.[7] The rationale for this decentralization of control over nursing homes and other facilities for the aged was improved coordination with social and home services, which traditionally have been financed and provided at the municipal level. To ensure a smooth transition, the Ministry of Social Affairs and Health developed a complex system of five-year shrinking subsidies from the counties to the municipalities; in effect, the municipalities (whose tax rate did not include funds for these residential services) are compensated by the counties (whose tax rate did). Despite some grumbling about the financial transfers (the counties claim they are too high, while the municipalities say they are too low), the overall re-structuring is deemed a success by Swedish policy makers.

Beyond the ÄDEL reform, there has been a prolonged debate in Sweden about the future structure of the health care system, tied to the activities of a Parliamentary Committee on Funding and Organization of Health Services and Medical Care (known in Swedish as "HSU 2000"). This Committee, established in 1992 by the then-sitting conservative government, was charged with recommending which of three designated health care models should be adopted: a reformed county council model, a primary care managed model or a compulsory public health insurance model. The Committee has held extensive hearings and its Expert Group has issued a preliminary report.[8] While some observers note that the national government is in practice following behind the county councils, and thus may find its options pre-empted by the time the recommendations become legislation, others see the national role as one of consolidation, laying out the direction for the health care system for the next several decades.

The Committee chose to hold its final report until after the September 1994 elections. All indications, however, are that it will adopt the least radical approach, the reformed county council model. This would entail two major structural changes: decentralization of all primary health care services to the municipal level; and consolidation of the 26 counties into 10 or 12 substantially larger units, which, in addition to managing the hospital system, could be merged with a separate, provincial system of national representation at the regional level *(länstyrelsen)* into a new, elected, regional parliament *(länsparliamentet)* with broad regional planning and development responsibilities. This new parliament would retain the right of counties to tax individual incomes, thus maintaining at both the regional and municipal level the link between direct financial responsibility and health services management.

REFORMS TO ALLOCATION MECHANISMS

Northern European countries have made a number of major reforms to the mechanisms by which taxes collected to finance health care are transferred to providers. Overall, the introduction of limited competitive incentives to what were command-and-control provider payment systems has become the single most important characteristic of the current reform era. Sweden and the UK initiated this process in 1990 and 1991, respectively, while Finland introduced major reform in 1993. Denmark, at the end of 1992, made the first of what will likely be substantial changes. With the exception of efforts to control pharmaceutical costs, which in the UK and Sweden, as elsewhere in the OECD, have been based on renewed regulatory controls (national formularies and/or reference pricing), most allocation-related reforms rely upon one or another competitive incentive derived from market-style notions of managing organizational behaviour.

United Kingdom

With the first wave of reforms in April 1991, the British government introduced two separate and conceptually contradictory means of provider payment. The first created managerially independent but still publicly owned and accountable hospitals labelled "self-governing trusts." These trusts would no longer receive fixed global budgets, but instead be required to compete for contracts in order to survive. The major source of contract business for the hospitals would continue to be the District Health Authority, which would be reconfigured as a purchaser of care. Thus this first restructured allocation mechanism sought to *separate* purchaser from provider, yet retain both within the *public* sector.

The second new allocation mechanism established fundholding GPs. Group practices of private physicians would be financially responsible for providing the patient not only with primary care, in return for a capitated fee, but also with elective inpatient services (up to £5,000 per inpatient stay). These fundholding GP groups (which were initially required to have 11,000 patients in the practice, later 7,000) were entitled to act as purchasers of some hospital services on behalf of their patients and were expected to negotiate contracts for care with whatever self-governing trust (or residual directly managed hospital) could provide the best price and quality. Thus this second restructured allocation mechanism sought to *combine* purchase and provision in the hands of a single entity that would be a strictly *private* enterprise.

These two mechanisms were designed to reach the same goal: better value for money.[9] The fact that they relied upon opposing conceptual frameworks — most likely a legacy of the frantic manner in which the Thatcher Administration cobbled the reform together at the last minute[10] — has thus far been viewed as only a minor theoretical annoyance. The UK government has announced that both models, which were extended to a third tranche of hospitals and GPs in April 1994, will in fact be expanded to cover all hospitals and GPs in the near future — in effect creating two new universal models for the British health care system.

Although British ministers have steadfastly maintained that there is no need to evaluate these reforms, independent critics have pointed to a number of dilemmas.[11] The reforms have not substantially reduced the numbers waiting for at least a year for elective procedures, and they have required substantial additional funds to cover the larger transaction costs of a price-based health market.[12] Patients have little say in where they are sent for inpatient care, the decision being made on predominantly financial grounds by whichever of the two purchasers, the District Health Authority or the fundholding GP group, controls their clinical fates. Perhaps most sensitively, there are concerns that the reforms, by encouraging fundholding GPs to get faster and/or better inpatient care for their patients, will serve to further reduce equity in a system already documented as having substantial equity problems.[13]

It remains to be seen whether the combination of trusts and fundholding practices can in fact generate enough efficiency to justify their economic and social costs. In 1992, 89 percent of contracts between District Health Authorities and hospital trusts were of a non-specific "block contract" character,[14] in which providers simply agree to provide clinical services as needed over a fixed period. This suggests that this particular allocation mechanism will require further development.

Sweden

In Sweden, the main payment mechanism for provider institutions is being shifted from a fixed annual budget to a combination of patient choice (consumer sovereignty) and negotiated contracts.

To accommodate this shift, an increasing number of county councils expect the provider institutions to act as public firms — that is, to be paid based on their productivity and performance.[15] Since 1991, patient choice has become integral to the Swedish system.[16] A patient can choose a hospital or health centre anywhere in the country. In turn, in a growing number of counties[17] the hospitals and health centres are paid by the volume of patients they attract. In Stockholm County, since January 1992, hospitals have been paid on a Diagnosis Related Group (DRG) basis, as have certain surgical units in an experimental sample of 10 hospitals nationwide.[18] One outcome of these measures (in combination with provider awareness of over-capacity of inpatient beds and concern about institutional survival) is that waiting lists for elective procedures are no longer than 12 weeks — a substantial achievement given that queues for a number of procedures were two years long in 1991.[19]

Another emphasis of Swedish reform has been the development of contract-based allocation mechanisms. These were introduced in 1990 and 1991, and now nearly all counties are at least in the process of developing a contract-based framework.[20] These arrangements are of two basic types. One involves splitting the existing public sector into two entities — purchasing and a grouping of provider institutions. The second decentralizes the purchasing function to a number of sub-county boards, which then are responsible for both administering the local primary care system and purchasing hospital services for the local population as needed.

While both formats involve a version of what the British refer to as a "purchaser-provider split," their role in the Swedish context is quite different. First, the purchasing boards typically are composed of elected local politicians directly accountable to their constituents. Hence the purchasing boards are intended to enhance local accountability, rather than undercut it as in the business model promoted in the UK. Second, these negotiated contracts can do no more than indicate patient volume. They co-exist with patient choice, and patients retain the right to go wherever they choose, regardless of where contracts are let.

It is interesting to note that, contrary to the assumptions of some health economists in the US, in all three large metropolitan areas in Sweden patient choice *per se* does *not* cost the counties appreciably more in expenditures of real revenues. Of course, in the Swedish context patient choice creates minimal costs because it is exercised within a fully publicly operated health system characterized by fixed expenditure ceilings and salaried physicians. Patient choice in the US, by contrast, is expensive because it exists in a health care system with no overall expenditure limits and fee-for-service payment for physicians — fee-for-service being notorious for raising costs in every health system in which it is found.

Third, in counties like Dalarna and Stockholm, which have adopted a system of decentralized sub-county boards, the entity that holds population responsibility and contracts for hospital services also directly administers the primary care system. In effect, this means a combining of functions that in the UK reform are split between district authority and fundholding GPs.

As the co-existence in some counties of patient choice and negotiated contracts suggests, some Swedish reforms seek to combine two apparently contradictory mechanisms of resource allocation. Thus far, patient choice and the principle "the money follows the patient" has been predominant, with negotiated contracts organized as "soft" contracts that establish treatment relationships, certain quality parameters and perhaps prices, but that do not guarantee a specified patient volume.[21] Stockholm County's Western District has sought to solve this dilemma by establishing networks of care that are of sufficiently high quality that patients will choose to be treated in those institutions with which the District has contracts.[22] It is not clear how these two different principles of provider payment will co-exist if contracts become more specific. It seems unlikely, however, that after finally gaining the right to choose their physician and site of treatment Swedish patients will easily let it be restricted or withdrawn.

In addition to county-led reforms concerning patient choice and negotiated contracts, in 1993 the conservative Swedish government introduced a major restructuring of the primary care system and how its physicians are paid. Every county was expected, by mid-1995, to transform its primary care centres — in which most physicians are salaried employees of the county —into a Danish- or British-style system of independent entrepreneurial GPs.[23] The national reform sought to override recent efforts by some counties to turn health centres into various types of "public firms" similar to the way in which hospitals have been organized. In Stockholm County, where the conservative-dominated county council had already begun to implement the legislation, concerns were voiced about its implications for the team approach to primary care, and for the future of preventive and population-based initiatives. There also were disputes with physicians about the appropriate annual patient capitation fee.[24]

Finland

The Finnish government embarked in January 1993 upon a major reform of the mechanism by which funds for health services are allocated.[25] Funding for the publicly operated health service system continues to be split more or less evenly between the national government and the 460 municipalities; however, the government has changed three crucial criteria upon which State monies are distributed through the municipalities to the health care providers.

In the previous system, the Ministry of Social Affairs and Health, in conjunction with the (now re-structured) National Board of Health, established a national plan for each budget year.[26] The plan stipulated exactly how many professional personnel each municipality could employ in its primary health centre and social services or in each hospital. (Hospitals and primary health centres are owned and operated by municipalities, either singly or in small federations.) National subsidies were then provided as a set percentage of salary of each approved employee, dependent upon the overall financial status of the municipality (subsidies ranged from 31 to 69 percent).

In the new system, national subsidies will be calculated not as a percentage of salary for approved personnel, but on the basis of number of citizens resident in the municipality, adjusted for age and sex. This change will be phased in over a five-year period. Moreover, as of 1993 funds are paid to municipalities in block grants, with a single lump-sum payment for all health and social services (including public housing and child care). This has created two new situations for the municipalities: they themselves decide how to allocate available revenues between health and a number of other municipal functions, and they themselves receive the revenues for hospital services — whereas under the former system these were paid directly to the hospital.

In sum, the Finnish reform — known as the Hiltunen Plan, for the Finance Ministry official who proposed it in 1989 — has three components: (1) a shift from position-based to a population capitation system of national subsidies, (2) lump-sum payments directly to the municipality and (3) a block-grant approach in which health funds are commingled with those of various social services. Viewed internationally, the Hiltunen measures are consistent with efforts elsewhere to decentralize health-related responsibilities to the lowest possible level in the public sector. In practice, they reflect the insistence of Finnish municipal officials that they be freed from the tight fiscal strait-jacket of the national plan.

The overall performance of the new subsidy system is not yet clear, in part due to the financial strictures that have accompanied the present severe contraction in the Finnish economy and the rise in unemployment to 20 percent. Payments to the municipalities for health and social services were noticeably lower in 1994 than in the previous year, and at least one municipality was reported in late 1993 to already be bankrupt.[27] As part of an ongoing discussion about how to shrink public expenditures, the issue of combining the national health insurance scheme (predominantly for privately delivered outpatient services) with the system of national and municipal financing for publicly operated health services is again being discussed.

Now that all revenues for the health system are held directly by Finland's 460 municipalities, local officials are being forced to develop a system of contracts by which to allocate revenues to hospitals. Thus far, they have generally adopted a Finnish version of block contracting, which in Finland, as in the UK, has been meaningful precisely because patients do not have the right to select their health centre or hospital. However, given that prior restrictions on public sector contracting with private providers were removed by the legislation that enacted the Hiltunen Plan, municipalities can be expected to introduce more specific cost and volume contracts with both public and private providers in the near future.

It should be noted that the contracting entity also directly manages the system of primary care providers. This is true both in Finland, where the contracting process is in municipal hands, and in those Swedish counties that have decentralized their purchasing function to sub-county (in some instances, municipality-congruent) political boards.

Not surprisingly, current experience is that the contracts that these purchasing entities take out with hospitals are heavily influenced by the chief physician of the local health centre. This has the advantage of allowing the primary care sector to define what hospital services are appropriate for its population and to have control over the funds paid to hospitals and hospital specialists for those services, while at the same time ensuring that the contracts are subject to the scrutiny of the local population. It is in this continuation of primary care control and public accountability that the Nordic approach differs from the system of private fundholding GPs in the UK.

Denmark

Current policy in Denmark is that major reform of its allocation mechanism is neither needed nor contemplated.[28] Nonetheless, three recent changes suggest that allocation mechanisms may eventually follow along in the Swedish direction.

One of these changes was initially developed by North Jutland County Council and was then introduced nationwide (and subsequently adopted in Sweden's ÄDEL reform). It requires that municipal social services accept an elderly inpatient within five days of notification that the patient has finished a course of treatment. This reform has had great success in both counties in removing "bed blockers" from inpatient beds.[29]

A second Danish reform was the introduction, in October 1992, of a patient's right to seek treatment at any hospital in the country (patients have always had the right to select their private primary care doctor).

The third reform was the adoption of a Swedish-style 100-day guarantee of treatment for a limited number of treatments with long queues. Hospitals in other counties are compensated by the county in which the patient resides according to a national set of rates originally developed for out-of-county emergency care. Thus far, there are no experiments with intra-county negotiated contracts; however, mounting financial pressures and continuing long waiting times[30] suggest that Danish counties will be closely watching the results of current contract-based reforms in Sweden and Finland.

PRODUCTION-SIDE REFORMS

Changes on the production side of Northern European health systems reflect institutional responses to newly introduced allocation mechanisms.

First, consistent with the introduction of competitive incentives such as negotiated contracts and patient choice of provider, hospitals in most Northern European countries are being transformed from directly administered public institutions into one or another type of independently managed public enterprise. Second, primary care physicians, to the degree that they had previously been salaried civil servants, are undergoing a reconfiguration of their payment system so that there will be a greater connection between productivity and income. Third — and perhaps most controversially — the UK, Sweden and Finland are all conducting experiments in which primary care political boards, centres or doctors are given control over a large segment of the inpatient and outpatient funds that their primary care patients are expected to spend. This section will review each of these major changes.

The most visible new competitive incentive on the production side of Northern European health systems concerns publicly operated hospitals. Institutions that were previously paid on a fixed global budget are being reconfigured as independent public enterprises, similar in structure to an airport or port authority. While they are still publicly owned and held publicly accountable for their overall performance, the hospitals are expected to attract a sufficient volume (through negotiated contracts and/or patient choice) to pay their personnel and expenses.

There are differences, of course, between the "self-governing trusts" in the UK and the "public firms" emerging in Sweden and Finland. British hospitals, for example, are managerially accountable to the national Department of Health, and for capital investment to the Treasury, while hospitals in Sweden are accountable to county councils and those in Finland to municipal governments. Nevertheless, the pattern is one of continued public ownership and strict controls over new capital — but with independent entrepreneurial management and with payment tied to productivity.

The second area of structural reform on the production side of health systems involves the payment structure for primary care physicians. In Sweden, physicians in some counties are being changed in status from civil servants in county-run primary health centres to independent entrepreneurs on the Danish or British GP model. In the case of Finland, most primary care physicians continue to work within the publicly run health centres; however, they are now organized on a small-area population responsibility basis and are being paid through a set of capitated arrangements. In both countries, primary care physicians are no longer salaried but are paid in some relationship to performance.

Third, at least three Northern European countries have developed mechanisms by which a substantial portion of revenue intended to purchase hospital care will be controlled by primary care physicians (the UK) and/or by political bodies linked to primary care (Sweden and Finland). These arrangements are designed to meet several interrelated objectives: to reduce unnecessary hospital referrals, to encourage higher quality and lower cost hospital services, to improve continuity of care and — to the extent that they can choose their primary care physician and/or contracting agent (in England and Sweden) — to give patients a degree of leverage in the decisions made about their hospital care. Here, too, the eventual allocation mechanism is the negotiated contract — in this instance between GP and/or primary care agent and hospital.

ON THE ROLE OF COMPETITIVE INCENTIVES

The current wave of reforms in Northern European health systems has been under way for three to five years. A number of proposals are now being implemented, and several of these have been in place long enough to support assessments of their progress to date.[31] It is therefore possible to sketch out patterns that can serve to characterize the reform process as a whole.

Reforms to the tax-financed health systems of the UK and the Nordic Countries are as important for what they have preserved as for what they have sought to change.[32] The reforms have understood the role of competitive mechanisms, and of market forces generally, as one that should reinforce rather than undercut traditional public sector objectives such as solidarity in health care financing and public accountability on the part of providers. While the meaning of these concepts varies from country to country — the British government, for example, understands accountability as predominantly financial, whereas the Swedes seek direct political as well as financial accountability — the pattern is nonetheless consistent. Competitive behaviour has been introduced in carefully calibrated doses on the production side of health systems — between hospitals, for example — in pursuit of institutional-level micro-efficiency in the areas of productivity, medical effectiveness and responsiveness to patients. These production-side competitive incentives have been supported and stimulated by allocation changes, typically by tying provider payment mechanisms (particularly for hospitals and GPs) to some standard of productivity.

One intriguing aspect of the reform process has been the different national decisions taken about the *type* of competitive incentives to adopt, particularly decisions about the balance between mechanisms that strengthen the hand of managers (negotiated contracts) and those that shift more decision making to patients (patient choice).

In the UK, in the primary care area, the fundholding GPs may have increased the ability of some individuals to choose in that they can select a fundholder that has a particular set of contracts and that consequently may have some leverage in hospital scheduling. But that is a marginal increment. Overall in the UK, patients have lost in terms of their power to choose, because District Health Authorities — i.e., managers — now hold specific contracts that tell patients where to obtain care, and patients do follow the money. In Sweden, patient choice has a dominant role and thus far none of the counties has interfered, in part because Swedes feel strongly about this issue. In Finland, the discussion on patient choice has not been engaged yet and patients do not have much choice within the public system. However, when Finnish patients are not happy with a non-choice, they tend to buy their way out, moving to the private sector for the service in question. This is one reason why Finland has a relatively large private sector, particularly in terms of ambulatory care.

The diversity of approaches reflects a difference in the objectives that health reforms are expected to achieve. In Sweden, a key policy objective has been the use of patient choice as a steering mechanism to alter patterns of resource allocation within the system. The British approach is to encourage the manager to gain more control. In effect, Sweden's reforms have sought to increase patient power while those in the UK have sought to optimize that of managers.

Northern European health care reform has not relied exclusively on competitive incentives. Strong public sector regulatory measures have been employed in the development of these new "planned markets,"[33] and, where necessary, in the introduction of command-and-control measures focussed on the quality and cost of services like reference pricing and various types of formularies for pharmaceutical drugs. Although it might appear counter-intuitive, competitive incentives have increased the need for regulation by the central government. National ministries of health are opening up their providers to competitive pressures and decentralizing day-to-day institutional decision-making powers, to either independently managed public sector organizations or (in the case of primary care reform in Sweden) new private entrepreneurs. This has generated pressure to establish a new range of national regulations concerning service standards and the monitoring and evaluation of characteristics such as access, quality and outcomes.[34] Such regulation is essential if governments are to make good on their guarantees of equal access for all citizens.

A key aspect of current reforms has been that competitive incentives in these tax-financed health systems have been limited almost exclusively to the public sector. Despite initial noises from conservative politicians about the advantages of mixed public-private markets, notably in the UK and Stockholm County, there have been few efforts to privatize existing institutions. Instead, emphasis has been placed on transforming them into independent public firms that stay within the public sector. Similarly, there has been little sustained interest among public purchasing agencies to contract private specialist physician and/or hospital services. In fact, in some quarters in both Sweden and the UK[35] it is felt that it may not even be necessary to introduce competitive incentives in the public sector in order to bring about the changes. Administrators in largely rural Älvsborg County, for instance, argue that they have achieved greater efficiency and more dramatic cost control through a continued command-and-control public sector model.[36] Overall, however, on the production and allocation side, the application of competitive incentives among publicly operated institutions — or "public competition"[37] — has been substantially more common in Northern Europe than have either a mixed public-private approach or the traditional command-and-control format.

Having discussed where competitive incentives are being used, it should be noted where they are *not*. None of these Northern European countries is using or is seeking to use competitive incentives on the finance side of their health systems. Conservative as well as social democratic governments retain publicly run, single-source financing structures, on the grounds of lower operating costs, better macroeconomic control and greater long-term organizational stability, as well as (for the Nordic Countries) to maintain solidarity and traditional welfare state values.

The pattern of Northern European use of competitive incentives should send a valuable message to policy makers in a number of other tax-financed systems in OECD countries currently reviewing their health sectors. It should be particularly instructive for decision makers in those systems financed by social insurance that are flirting with the idea of introducing competitive incentives, like the Netherlands and Germany, and also for American proponents of competitive health financing strategies such as managed competition.

1. Finland's 1990–91 fall in its overall GDP of some 10 percent, due to a dramatic reduction in trade with the former Soviet Union, resulted in Finnish health expenditures as a percentage of GDP rising above the OECD average in 1991.

2. C. Ham, R. Robinson and M. Benzeval, *Health Check: Health Policy in an International Perspective* (London: King's Fund Institute, 1990).

3. Richard B. Saltman, "A Conceptual Overview of Recent Health Care Reforms," *European Journal of Public Health* (forthcoming 1994).

4. J. Higgins, *The Business of Medicine: Private Health Care in Britain* (London: Macmillan Education, 1988).

5. SPRI, *The Reform of Health Care in Sweden* (Stockholm: SPRI, 1992).

6. Finnish Ministry of Health, "Health Reform in Finland," country chapter submitted for Phase II of the OECD project on Health Reform, Helsinki, 1993.

7. SPRI, *The Reform of Health Care in Sweden.*

8. Ministry of Health and Social Affairs, *Three Models for Health Care Reform in Sweden,* Report from the Expert Group to the Committee on Funding and Organization of Health Services and Medical Care (HSU 2000), Stockholm, 1993.

9. R. Robinson and J. Le Grand (eds.), *Evaluating the NHS Reforms* (London: King's Fund Institute, 1994).

10. Ham, Robinson and Benzeval, *Health Check: Health Policy in an International Perspective.*

11. C. Ham, "Health Care Reform: The Difficulties of Controlling Spending at the Macro Level while Promoting Efficiency at the Micro Level," *British Medical Journal,* Vol. 386 (May 1993), pp. 1223–24.

12. C. Smee, "Self-Governing Trusts and Budget-Holding GPs: The British Experience," in Richard B. Saltman and Casten von Otter (eds.), *Implementing Planned Markets in Health Care: Balancing Social and Economic Responsibility* (Buckingham, UK and Philadelphia: Open University Press, forthcoming 1995).

13. M. Whitehead, *The Health Divide* (London: Penguin, 1988); and "Is It

Fair? Evaluating the Equity Implications of the NHS Reforms," in Robinson and Le Grand, *Evaluating the NHS Reforms,* pp. 208–42.

14. Smee, "Self-Governing Trusts and Budget-Holding GPs."

15. S.-E. Bergman, "Purchaser-Provider Systems in Sweden," paper presented to the Scottish Comparative Study Tour, Gävle, September 1, 1993.

16. Richard B. Saltman, "Patient Choice and Patient Empowerment in Northern European Health Systems: A Conceptual Framework," *International Journal of Health Services,* Vol. 24, no. 2 (1994), pp. 201–30.

17. Although the national government sets the framework for the Swedish health system, each of the 26 county councils is legally independent in how it administers the health care system. Each county makes its own decisions on organizational reform, resulting in the perception that, organizationally speaking, Sweden has not one but 26 different publicly operated health care systems. See Richard B. Saltman and Casten von Otter, *Planned Markets and Public Competition: Strategic Reform in Northern European Health Systems* (Buckingham, UK, and Philadelphia: Open University Press, 1992).

18. A. Anell, "Implementing Planned Markets in Health-Care Services: The Swedish Case," in Saltman and von Otter (eds.), *Implementing Planned Markets.*

19. T. Malm, personal communication, February 23, 1994.

20. Bergman, "Purchaser-Provider Systems in Sweden."

21. For a discussion of hard as against soft contracts see Casten von Otter, "The Application of Market Principles to Health Care," in D. J. Hunter (ed.), *Paradoxes of Competition for Health* (Leeds: Nuffield Institute, 1991), pp. 13–22.

22. Malm, personal communication.

23. Anell, "Implementing Planned Markets in Health-Care Services."

24. The Social Democrats regained power in the September 1994 elections. They are likely to stop if not reverse much of this primary care re-organization. Some county councils, for example the Centre Party-led administration in Gotland, had already announced that they think their existing health centre-based primary care service is functioning well and that in any event they would not introduce the new "house

doctor" system. G. Berleen, personal communication, May 6, 1994.

25. Finnish Ministry of Health, "Health Reform in Finland."

26. Richard B. Saltman, "National Planning for Locally Controlled Health Systems: The Finnish Experience," *Journal of Health Politics, Policy and Law,* Vol. 13, no. 1 (Spring 1988), pp. 27–51.

27. M. Lehto, personal communication, October 1, 1993.

28. Danish Ministry of Health, "Health Care in Denmark," country chapter submitted for Phase II of the OECD project on Health Reform, Copenhagen, 1992.

29. See Danish Ministry of Health, "Health Care in Denmark."

30. P. Lorin, "Strid om operationsköer," *Landstingsvarlden* 7/94, 1994, p. 23.

31. See Howard Glennerster, M. Matsaganis and P. Owens, *A Foothold for Fundholding* (London: King's Fund Institute, 1992); Smee, "Self-Governing Trusts and Budget-Holding GPs"; E. Jonsson, *Konkurrens inom sjukvarden: vad säger forskningen om effekterna?* (Stockholm: SPRI, 1993); and Anell, "Implementing Planned Markets in Health-Care Services."

32. Richard B. Saltman, "Recent Health Policy Initiatives in the Nordic Countries," *Health Care Financing Review,* Vol. 13, no. 4 (Summer 1992), pp. 157–66.

33. Saltman and von Otter, *Planned Markets and Public Competition.*

34. Saltman, "A Conceptual Overview of Recent Health Care Reforms."

35. Ham, "Health Care Reform."

36. P.-O. Brogren, personal communication, February 6, 1994.

37. Saltman and von Otter, *Planned Markets and Public Competition.*

W Y N A N D   P .   M .   M .   V A N   D E   V E N

A N D   F R E D E R I K   T .   S C H U T

The Dutch Experience

with Internal Markets

Introduction

In 1988 the Dutch government embarked on a radical reform of its health care system. This undertaking was inspired by the Enthoven Consumer Choice Health Plan[1] and was based on the recommendations of the Dekker Commission. The system proposed at that time can be described as a national health insurance scheme based on regulated competition. The reforms represent a transition from government-regulated cartels to government-regulated competition among insurers and providers of care, whereby competing insurers selectively contract with competing providers. Insurers therefore function as third-party purchasers of care. Since 1989, when step-by-step implementation of the reforms was begun, a number of major changes have taken place and new problems have emerged.

We will describe the main thrust of the reforms and then go on to outline the progress made so far: the goals that have and have not been reached and the obstacles that have arisen. We will then discuss a major issue in a competitive health insurance market (or third-party purchase of care) with a regulated premium structure: cream skimming, or preferred risk selection — selection by the insurer or third-party purchaser of those insureds for whom the costs are expected to be lower than the revenues.

HEALTH CARE REFORM IN THE NETHERLANDS

Why Such Radical Reforms?

The Dutch health care system, despite the predominance of private ownership, is heavily regulated by government.

During the period 1960–80, health expenditures as a percentage of GDP doubled, from 3.9 to 8.0 percent. In order to control this rise, a considerable amount of government regulation has been introduced, especially since the mid-1970s. During the 1980s, health expenditures as a percentage of GDP remained relatively stable, mainly as a result of government-imposed restraints on hospital capacity (introduced in the 1970s), global budgeting of hospitals (1983), manpower planning, regulation of nurses' salaries and detailed regulation of volume, price and productive capacity. So one may wonder why the government chose to embark on such radical reforms.

In 1988, the centre-right coalition government put forth the following four reasons for reforming the health care system.[2]

1. The *uncoordinated financing structure* of health care and social welfare (social work, homes for the aged and family assistance programmes) was an impediment to cost-effective substitution of different forms of health care delivery. Closely interrelated forms of delivery were frequently artificially separated by multiple financing mechanisms and complex regulations. For instance:

- Hospital and GP care was covered by "sickness" funds or private health insurers.
- Home care was financed as part of a compulsory national health insurance scheme for catastrophic risks (the Exceptional Medical Expense Act, or AWBZ).
- Family assistance programmes were covered by private payments as well as from the national budget.
- Social work was covered by private payments as well as from the municipal budget.
- The financing of nursing home care was based on the AWBZ.
- Homes for the aged were heavily subsidized from the national budget.

There were strict regulations governing the nature of care, the institution that is to deliver the care, the point of delivery, and so on. Furthermore, the financing system was oriented toward the institution rather than the function (e.g., rehabilitation centre *versus* rehabilitation services). In sum, the government concluded that the combination of multiple financing and complex regulations served to impede efficient substitution of care.

2. The Dutch health care system was suffering from a *lack of incentives for efficiency.* There were few financial incentives in this regard for the parties involved: the producers, consumers and insurers of care. The financing system was such that in many cases economic, efficient behaviour was financially punished, while non-economic, inefficient behaviour was financially rewarded. Therefore, transformation of the present financing system was a necessary condition for improved efficiency.

3. *Detailed regulation had negative results.* According to the government, many of the problems in the health care system were a result of complex legislation and detailed regulation:

■ The very detailed regulation of capacity planning in health care had proved to be unworkable. This failure was a result of the complexity of the planning process, the large number of parties involved and their conflicting interests and the lack of clarity of the regulations (many rapid changes and inconsistencies with other forms of regulation).

■ The relationship between planning and financing presented a major problem. A crucial question was whether planning should precede or follow financing. In the existing system, planning and financing decisions were made separately, causing many problems; none of the parties involved were fully responsible for the consequences of their decisions.

■ The centrally regulated system of remunerating providers was an impediment to flexibility and efficient allocation. The nationwide fee schedule did not take into account specific regional or local circumstances. Since the early 1980s, the remuneration system had been a source of conflict between government and health care providers.

4. There were *several problems with the health insurance system.* All employees (and their families) earning less than 56,000 guilders (about US$30,000) annually were compulsorily insured by one of the 20 sickness funds. This also held true after retirement. A limited number of

civil servants had their own mandatory scheme. The remainder of the population (about 34 percent), mainly self-employed and high-income persons, had the option of buying coverage, choosing from among the 40 private health insurers operating in the Netherlands. Finally, a compulsory national health insurance scheme (AWBZ) covered the entire population against catastrophic risks, such as hospital care exceeding one year, long-term nursing home care and long-term institutional care for the mentally and physically handicapped. Without going into detail, the many problems of the Dutch system related to the existence of different insurance schemes with different premium structures and to the effects of an unregulated competitive market for private health insurance.[3]

In 1990, the new centre-left coalition government endorsed the above arguments, stressing the failure of detailed regulation to control volume, prices, and productive capacity. It saw as the major cause of this failure the fact that only government was responsible for cost containment. All other parties — providers, insurers and insureds — could oppose regulation without committing themselves in any way. The government expressed serious doubt that, in a system under which it is the only braking factor, cost could be maintained, in the long run, without jeopardizing quality. From that government's point of view, therefore, the sharing of responsibility for cost containment with providers, insurers, and insureds was a major purpose of the reform.

The Proposal

In March 1988 the government proposed a market-oriented reform of the health sector.[4] This proposal, which was based on the recommendations of the Dekker Commission (March 1987), was endorsed by Parliament in the autumn of 1988.

In 1990 the main points of the proposal were adopted by the new government.[5] Since that time the reform has been referred to as the Simons Plan, for the Secretary of State for Health, Hans Simons. Although the 1990 proposal is essentially the same as the 1988 version, the vocabulary reflects the social democratic background of the Secretary of State for Health. Key words found in the earlier proposal by the centre-right cabinet are "competition," "market" and "incentives." In the 1990 version these are replaced by terms like "shared responsibility between parties," "consumer choice" and "decentralization." Nevertheless, the 1990 Simons Plan is very similar to the 1987 Dekker Plan.

The proposed system can be best characterized as compulsory national health insurance ("basic insurance") based on regulated competition. Direct government control over prices and productive capacities will make way for regulated competition among insurers and among health care providers. Price cartels and regional cartels formed as a result of anti-competitive government regulation and self-regulation will be broken down. The basic benefits package will be comprehensive: nearly all non-catastrophic risks (hospital care, physician services, drugs, physiotherapy, some dental care), catastrophic risks (nursing home care, long-term institutional care for the mentally and physically handicapped), and health care related to social welfare (homes for the elderly). Together, these benefits account for about 95 percent of health expenditures (including social welfare-related health). Not included in the basic benefits package is "supplemental" care such as cosmetic surgery and homeopathic medicine. In addition, the population must pay 10 percent of the total expenditures in the form of user fees.

According to the proposal, all individuals will receive a subsidy to purchase their compulsory insurance from one of the competing insurers.[6] The subsidy will be paid by a Central Fund directly to the qualified insurer chosen by the insured. The Central Fund will be financed by mandatory income-related premiums collected by the tax department. Qualified insurers will not be able to refuse any insured in their area of operation and must abide by other pro-competitive regulations. The maximum contract period will be two years, so that at least once every two years the consumer will have the opportunity to change insurers. The subsidy per individual will be independent of the chosen insurer and will be equal to the expected per capita health care costs within the risk group to which the insured belongs, minus a fixed amount that will be the same for everyone. The deficit created by this deducted fixed amount will be met by a flat-rate premium paid by the insured directly to the insurer of choice. Figure 1 provides an overview of the proposed financing system.

An insurer will be obliged to quote the same flat rate to every insured who chooses the same contract, so that the insurer's revenues will come from the risk-adjusted per capita payment from the Central Fund supplemented by the flat-rate premium paid by the insured. The difference between actual costs and the risk-adjusted payment will not be the same for all insurers and will be reflected in the flat-rate premium quoted by

Figure 1

Proposed Health Care Financing Scheme in the Netherlands*

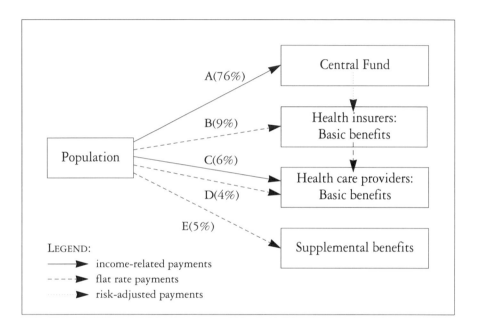

* According to the current (1993) proposals the basic benefits package should comprise 95 percent of total health care expenditures (i.e., A+B+C+D=95 percent). Two other restrictions are that 82 percent of the total health care expenditures should be covered by income-related payments (A+C=82 percent) and that (at least) 15 percent of the total health care expenditures should be paid directly to the provider of care (C+D+E=15 percent). Because the current income-related direct payments (primarily for institutional long-term care) are assumed to remain six percent of total health care costs (C=six percent), the size of the payments as a percentage of total health care costs are as given in the figure.

SOURCE: Ministry of Health, Letter to Parliament, 5 June 1992, Tweede Kamer 1991-92, 22393 (20) (Note "Modernisering zorgsector: Weloverwogen verder"), SDU, The Hague, 1992.

the competing insurers. This will create the incentive for insurers to be efficient.

The insurer will be expected to function as intermediary between consumer and provider. Insurers and providers will be largely free to negotiate the terms of the contract. The law will describe the standardized basic benefits package not in terms of institutions like hospitals or nursing homes, but rather in terms of types of care. For instance, the entitlements of the insureds will no longer be described as "services provided by licensed rehabilitation centres" but as "rehabilitation services." Any provider meeting certain standards of quality will be able to offer these services, which will greatly increase the possibilities for cost-effective substitution. Insurers will be allowed to selectively contract with providers and to offer different contracts, as long as they cover every type of care as described by law. The insurance contracts will be different forms of the standardized benefits package and may vary only with respect to the *list of contracted providers of care* and with respect to the *conditions* that must be fulfilled in order for costs to be covered (for instance, whether a referral slip from a GP is required for reimbursement of a specialist consultation fee).

This flexibility in the description of the standardized package should pave the way for alternative health care delivery and insurance arrangements, such as Health Maintenance Organizations (HMOs) and Preferred Provider Organizations (PPOs). Consumers will be free to choose among insurers, selecting whatever form of standardized benefits package best suits them. Some people will prefer a traditional health insurance contract with free choice of provider, while others may opt for a limited provider plan with a lower premium. Furthermore, the premium will reflect the efficiency and cost-generating behaviour of the contracted providers. It is expected that this will create an environment in which:

- Insureds are rewarded for choosing efficient insurers and cost-effective providers.
- Providers are rewarded for providing care effectively and efficiently.
- Insurers, acting as intermediaries between insured consumers and contracted providers, are motivated to contract efficient providers and to carry out market research in order to determine consumer preferences.

What Has and Has Not Been Realized

The 1988 proposal called for the reform to be in place by the end of 1992. In 1990, the deadline was extended by three years. In mid-1994, however, it is clear that this schedule was far too optimistic. In looking at the two key elements of the reform — basic insurance and regulated competition — we may conclude that as of 1994 neither of these has become reality. The prospects of seeing the reform fully realized are minimal. Nevertheless, in the early 1990s the following steps were taken toward a market-oriented system of health care:

- Since 1993, sickness funds have been receiving a partially *risk-adjusted capitation payment* from the Central Fund. In addition, each insured pays a flat-rate premium to his or her sickness fund (in 1994, about 10 percent of total sickness fund expenditures — i.e., about 200 guilders [US$120] per person yearly). Each sickness fund is free to determine its own flat-rate premium. (In 1994 these premiums are nearly all the same, as we shall see.) Those who are eligible for social security benefits (e.g., disabled and unemployed persons) receive a fixed cash sum to help pay the flat-rate premium. They nevertheless still have an incentive to choose, *ceteris paribus,* an inexpensive health insurance plan. The main points of the proposed financing system (see figure 1) have therefore been introduced into the sickness fund sector, which represents 62 percent of the population. This implies a radical change. During the period 1941–91 all sickness funds received full reimbursement for their medical expenditures. Therefore sickness funds are being transformed from administrative bodies into risk-bearing enterprises.

- As of 1994, sickness funds have the option to *selectively contract* with physicians and pharmacists. This too represents a radical change. Since 1941, sickness funds had a legal obligation to contract any provider in their area of operation who so wished it.

- Since 1992, sickness funds and private health insurers have been free to negotiate *lower fees* than those officially approved by government. An agency representing associations of providers, sickness funds and insurers sets the maximum fee according to government guidelines or directives. During the period 1982–92 it was an economic offence to charge higher or lower fees than those officially approved. It is expected that other

102

remuneration structures will in future be allowed, including capitation, withholds and bonuses, such as those in HMOs.

■ In 1992, sickness funds were permitted to extend their regional operating area and to include members in other parts of the country. In the previous decades it was practically impossible for them to do so because permission was usually not granted. Now almost all sickness funds operate *nationwide.*

■ In 1992, several private health insurance companies obtained permission to establish a new sickness fund, which suggests *open entry to the sickness fund market.* During the period 1941–91 no new sickness fund had been established (except through merger).

■ As of 1992, sickness fund members have the option to choose another sickness fund at least every two years. Every sickness fund must accept every eligible applicant. This could create competition among sickness funds based on the flat-rate premium, quality, contracted providers, service, responsiveness and reputation.

■ Since 1992, GPs have been *free to practise* wherever they want. Previously a municipal licence was required to set up a practice. The decision as to whether a new licence was available was dependent upon the number of GPs per capita in the municipality. If a licence was available, a profile of the desired characteristics of the GP was prepared and candidates could apply for the position in an open procedure.

We may conclude that these legislative changes represent important steps toward market-oriented health care and can be expected to fundamentally change the functioning and organization of the entire Dutch health care system. In our opinion the point-of-no-return has already passed. For *non-catastrophic risks* the changes are moving both the insurance and provision of health care to a system of "regulated competition." This is especially true since the changes have been supported by both a centre-left and a centre-right government. For these types of care, there is no turning back to the old regulatory regime.

The Effects So Far

It is much too early to fully evaluate the reforms, for the following reasons:

1. The legislative changes cannot be expected to have a great effect in the short term. Health care is like an oil tanker at full speed: it cannot

be turned around immediately.

2. Sickness funds, which play a key role in the reform process, have a 50-year history as regional administrative bodies and cannot be expected to become entrepreneurial, risk-bearing, consumer-oriented organizations overnight. Their first reaction to the pro-competitive measures was to engage in defensive mergers and to form (or, better, to continue with) various kinds of territorial and price cartels in order to eliminate or mitigate competition. Not surprisingly, in the first open enrolment period (in 1992) few insureds switched sickness funds. However, since the market has been opened for (competing) private health insurers, the cartel behaviour of the funds (e.g., forming agreements regarding premiums and acquisition of new members) has been substantially altered. Therefore, modest competition among funds can be expected.

3. Because of imperfections in the system of risk-adjusted capitation payments, sickness funds were held responsible in 1993 and 1994 for only three percent of the difference between their actual expenditures in 1993 and the normative expenditure level on which the risk-adjusted capitation payments are based. The remaining 97 percent of their expenses is still reimbursed retroactively (independently of the level of their flat-rate premium). This is another reason why all sickness funds have nearly the same flat-rate premium in 1994. It is the government's intention to increase the risk-bearing percentage for sickness funds while also improving the payment formula.

4. Despite these changes, a substantial element of the old regulatory regime is still in force — with respect to hospital budgeting and planning, for example. This hinders the development of innovative initiatives.

Nonetheless, the following effects of the reforms are worth mentioning:

- As a result of the discussion about a more market-oriented system, in the past few years we have seen a huge increase in activity around quality improvement and quality assurance. Several national conferences have been held on the subject, attended by official representatives of physicians, hospitals, insurers and consumers. The GP association has developed some 50 protocols for recurring medical complaints. Specialists are organizing quality assurance site visits to hospitals. Dentists are developing protocols. Medical associations are developing systems of re-registration (such as every five years) or re-certification. In the last three years there has been more activity concerning quality assurance and quality improvement than in the previous 20.

The driving force behind all this is probably the idea that quality will be the major issue in a competitive system. The prime interest, next to price, of the insurers, who (selectively) contract providers, will be quality and service, because that is what their insureds are interested in. Providers might also fear that if they themselves do not develop quality criteria, then the insurers will.

■ The early 1990s have seen increasing investment in cost-accounting systems by hospitals and other institutions. Most institutions are in the process of gradual transition from input to output pricing. At present, most prices in health care are administrative and bear no relation to the real costs of the services provided. These administrative prices provide misleading signals to all parties. Information about the nature and real costs of the various services is crucial to survival in a competitive market — to prevent providers from selling products below cost (i.e., at a loss) and so that insurers will buy care prudently and make the appropriate tradeoff between substitutes.

■ Since the early 1990s, the internal structure of the sickness funds has been totally reorganized as they prepare for their role as intermediary between consumer and provider in a competitive environment. As administration-oriented chief executives retire (some taking early retirement), they are being replaced by entrepreneurial, market-oriented managers. Service to fund members has been improved, by such measures as better hours and mobile offices. In the previous decades, when sickness funds enjoyed a regional monopoly, there was no need for such modification.

■ In anticipation of the proposed elimination of the difference between sickness fund insureds and privately insureds, there has been an integration of sickness funds and private insurers in the form of mergers, holding companies, etc. Each party has its own reasons for this.

Sickness funds hope to compensate for their lack of experience in marketing, actuarial calculation and entrepreneurship in a competitive environment. Furthermore, they fear that private health insurers have a competitive advantage because of their better image, because they sell group insurance and because they combine health insurance with other products (such as life, property and automobile insurance) and other financial services ("one-stop shopping").

A reason for private health insurers to integrate with sickness funds is to sell — via health insurance — other insurance products and financial services. (In health insurance there is frequent contact between insurer and insured, which gives the insurer the opportunity to sell other products.) Another advantage of integration for private insurers is that because the membership of sickness funds is regionally concentrated the insurers gain bargaining power at the regional level. Finally, integration offers private insurers the opportunity to benefit from the greater experience of the sickness funds in contracting with health care providers.

Industry observers expect that, as a result of these consolidations, within a few years there will be only 10 to 15 national chains of health insurers, serving a population of some 15 million.

■ The early 1990s have been years of innovation. For example, sickness funds have broken the price cartel of some medical-device suppliers; subsequently, prices have gone down by a quarter to a third. Insurers are developing mail-order firms as an alternative method of distributing pharmaceuticals. Many kinds of electronic data interchange (EDI) projects are being developed, to improve cooperation among providers and between providers and insurers.

■ Finally, consumer and patient organizations are increasing their activities. Consumer groups are educating the public about health insurance and the sickness funds. Consumer guides are publishing articles on health care. Hundreds of patient organizations have formed a national federation in order to become an effective interest group.

Reasons for the Slow Progress

Although implementation of the reforms is far behind schedule, from a historic point of view radical changes have taken place within a relatively short period of time. Take, for example, abolition of the contract obligation for sickness funds. The early decades of this century saw a long-standing conflict between physicians and sickness funds over whether sickness funds should have the option to selectively contract with physicians. Ultimately the physicians won, and from 1941 to 1991 sickness funds were legally obliged to enter into a uniform contract with each physician established in their area of operation. Though creating the opportunity for selective contracting is not the same as putting it into practice, it does represent a fundamental change.

Anyone familiar with the history of Dutch health care policy would have foreseen that the government's schedule was far too optimistic. On the other hand, if it had announced a more realistic time frame, such as 10 to 15 years, it is unlikely that any of the above changes would have taken place. As we have seen, the threat of competition has generated an enormous transformation in the conduct of all parties.

What are the reasons for the slow progress of the reforms? At least four can be identified.

1. There has been *resistance from interest groups* with powerful lobbies. Dutch health policy is characterized by a diffuse decision-making structure without a clear-cut centre of power. Hence, the government cannot impose changes without the consent of major interest groups such as associations of physicians, health insurers, employers and employees.[7] The *employers* oppose the Simons Plan because they fear the government will pay more attention to compulsory national health insurance with a broad benefits package, which would increase total health care costs (because of moral hazard), than to cost containment and efficiency. Because the premiums are partly paid by employers, increases in health expenditures would increase their labour costs and thereby weaken their international market position. The *insurers* oppose the Simons Plan because they strongly oppose a system of risk-adjusted capitation payments from the Central Fund and other government regulation that reduces their entrepreneurial freedom. The *physicians* oppose it because they find the functional description of the benefits package too general, leaving too much room for competition among providers of care.

2. The chosen implementation strategy has triggered growing *political opposition*. The Dutch government is traditionally composed of coalitions of at least two parties. The term of government is four years at maximum, which is far too short a period to implement comprehensive reforms. As a consequence, viable proposals must be reasonably acceptable to all major parties. From a political point of view, the two key elements of the reforms are well balanced. The basic insurance is attractive

to the left wing; regulated competition is attractive to the right wing. This political balance probably explains why both a centre-right and a centre-left coalition cabinet supported the reforms. Because of the complexity of the reforms, they must be implemented step by step, but such an approach itself introduces a new complexity. In order to be politically acceptable, each step must be just as balanced as the whole reform proposal. The politicians did not perceive it this way. The right wing, supported by the employers, strongly opposed certain of the steps because in their opinion more emphasis was put on implementation of the basic insurance than on cost containment.

There is another political issue: the introduction of basic insurance is likely to generate negative income-redistribution effects for relatively young and healthy middle-class people with private health insurance, because they will be subsidizing the poor and the unhealthy by paying an income-related premium instead of the present, considerably lower, risk-related premium.[8]

3. There is *no urgent need for reform.* In a sense, reorganization of the health care system anticipates the "luxury" problems of the next century: advanced medical technology, an ageing population and an expected increase in the health care share of the GDP. From a macroeconomic point of view, we can afford step-by-step reform.

4. The *technical complexity* of the reforms has been seriously underestimated. Several problems relate to the process of implementation, such as coordination of overlapping and sometimes inconsistent regulations, both old and new, avoidance of substantial negative wealth effects for parts of the population and fine tuning with complex European Community regulations. Another concerns the content and appropriate definition of the benefits that should be covered by the basic insurance. In addition, the problem of maintaining a viable competitive health care system should be addressed, which requires the development and implementation of an effective anti-cartel policy in health care.[9]

Probably the most vexing issue, however, relates to the proposed role of the insurer as a third-party purchaser of health care on behalf of the consumer. The question is how to prevent *cream skimming* in a competitive health insurance market in which insurers receive a risk-adjusted capitation payment.

We will concentrate on this problem, because it is not, like most of the others, specific to the Dutch reforms. Cream skimming is universal. It might be found in any competitive market for health insurance (or third-party purchasing of health care)[10] with a regulated premium structure.

CREAM SKIMMING

A key aspect of government regulation in the reformed Dutch health care system is determination of the risk-adjusted capitation payments the insurers receive from the Central Fund. The risk-adjusted payment per insured is dependent on the risk category to which the insured belongs. Since 1993, all sickness funds in the Netherlands receive such payments for most non-catastrophic risks (hospital care, physician services, drugs, physiotherapy, some dental care). In 1993 the age and gender of the insured were the risk factors used to adjust per capita payments. However, these risk categories appear to be much too heterogeneous. Sickness funds that have relatively unhealthy insureds per age-gender group receive payments that are too low. For example, the Amsterdam regional sickness fund claims that in Amsterdam there are, in each age-gender group, relatively high proportions of AIDS patients, drug addicts and people in low socio-economic groups, who are relatively unhealthy.

A major disadvantage of heterogeneous risk categories is that cream skimming may be very advantageous to the insurer. By cream skimming we mean selection by the insurer of "preferred risks" — i.e., those insureds for whom the insurer considers the risk-adjusted per capita payment to be far above the expected cost level. If age and gender are the only risk adjusters, cream skimming can be very profitable. On the basis of a previous study[11] we can conclude that the 10 percent of the population with the greatest non-catastrophic health expenditures (hospitals, physicians, pharmaceuticals) in any year can be predicted to have per capita expenditures four years later that are on average nearly double the per capita expenditures within their age-gender group. Based on its own claims records, therefore, each insurer can easily distinguish high-risk individuals.[12]

The adverse effects of cream skimming are threefold.

1. For the chronically ill, access to good health care may be hindered. Insurers will try to attract preferred risks and deter non-preferred risks. If the capitation payment system does not adequately compensate for health status, insurers might prefer not to contract with providers

who have a reputation for treating patients with AIDS, cancer, diabetes or high blood pressure, for instance, because they will not want to cover patients who are attracted by these providers.

2. In the case of an insufficiently refined payment system, *efficient* insurers may be driven out of the market by *inefficient* insurers who are successful at cream skimming.

3. Whilst individual insurers can gain by cream skimming, they merely shift the costs to others, so there is no social gain. In fact, because of the costs involved in the process of cream skimming, there can only be social losses. In sum, cream skimming is counter-productive with respect to the supposedly positive effects of competition: improved quality and efficiency of care and increased responsiveness to consumer preferences.

Lessons that can be learned from the Dutch experience with risk-adjusted capitation payments relate to several misunderstandings that have confused the debate in the Netherlands over the past five years.

One misunderstanding, especially among the civil servants responsible for designing the capitation payment system, was that age, gender and region would explain a large proportion of the variance in health care expenditure. If this were true, a capitation system based on these three risk adjusters alone would do a fairly good job. However, these risk factors are poor predictors of *individual* health expenditures and account for no more than two or three percent of the variance in individual expenditures[13] — i.e., between 10 and 20 percent of the *predictable* variance.[14] This misunderstanding may serve to explain this government decision: "For the time being the starting point is a *global* capitation formula."[15]

A second misunderstanding that has confused the debate is that a refinement of the capitation formula (i.e., extension of the capitation formula with a comprehensive set of relevant risk factors) would reduce market forces, and that eventually it would lead to a system of full reimbursement of all costs, thereby removing the insurers' incentive for efficiency. This false argument has been put forward often by actuaries and representatives of commercial insurers, who have a clear financial interest in a global capitation formula because of the relatively good health status of their insureds, and by politicians and top civil servants.[16] The flaw in this reasoning is the implicit assumption that differences in individual expenditures can be *fully predicted*. However, by far the largest part (at least 80 percent) of the difference in *individual* expenditures is unpredictable. Furthermore, a refined capitation payment would not remove the insurer's incentive for efficiency because, given a group of insureds, an insurer can influence the actual costs but not the prospectively determined capitation amount.[17] Therefore, each reduction in the actual costs will be fully reflected in the insurer's surplus.

A third misunderstanding is that commercial (risk-rated) re-insurance could solve the problem of cream skimming. The fallacy of this reasoning is as follows: the insurer must pay a risk-related premium to the commercial re-insurer. Therefore, the expected costs of a "bad risk" for the insurer will be the same (or even higher because of the loading fee included in the re-insurance premium). So, voluntary risk-rated re-insurance does not reduce the insurer's incentive to cream skim. Mandatory community-rated re-insurance, however, may help reduce this incentive.[18]

A major lesson of the Dutch reforms is that a system of sufficiently refined risk-adjusted capitation payments is a *necessary* condition for the success of such reforms.

In 1993 the payments to sickness funds were dependent on age and gender only. In order to reduce the disadvantages of an insufficiently refined payment system, the government introduced a system of risk sharing between the sickness funds and the Central Fund. In 1993–94 an individual sickness fund is responsible for only three percent of the difference between actual expenses and predicted expenses based on age and gender. However, as long as the remaining 97 percent is reimbursed retroactively the government prefers to retain most of the old tools for cost containment (although some fundamental changes have been made, as we have seen). Sickness funds, in turn, reproach government for providing them with financial risks without giving them the tools for cost containment. This vicious circle can be broken only by introducing a sufficiently refined payment system.

Therefore, a workable system of sufficiently refined risk-adjusted capitation payments is a *necessary* condition for reaping the fruits of a competitive health insurance market with a regulated premium structure.

On the basis of research findings[19] we are optimistic about the *technical* possibilities of finding a sufficiently refined capitation payment formula for *non-catastrophic* risks. However, the implementation of such a system requires considerable effort in the way of data collection, research and administration. In the first five years of reform the Dutch government has severely under-estimated these issues.

We cannot draw any conclusions about the technical (im)possibility of finding a sufficiently refined capitation payment formula for *catastrophic* risks such as long-term nursing home care and long-term institutional care for the mentally and physically handicapped. Age and gender, together with straightforward indicators like mental or physical handicap, are likely to yield higher proportions of predicted variance for individual catastrophic expenditures than for non-catastrophic expenditures; however, the *maximum* predictable variance is probably also much higher for catastrophic than for non-catastrophic expenditures. As far as we know, no empirical study has been carried out on risk-adjusted capitation payment formulas for catastrophic risks dealing with such questions as which risk adjusters should be included and the potential expected losses and profits for several sub-groups of insureds per set of risk adjusters. In the Netherlands, the relevant data required to carry out even an explorative study in this area are still lacking.

CONCLUSION AND DISCUSSION

Technical and Political Complexities

We have presented an overview of five years of market-oriented reform of the Dutch health care system. Although major changes have already been carried out, the implementation process will take much longer than the five years projected by the government; this because of resistance from interest groups and because of the technical and political complexity of the reforms.

There are technical problems to be solved. For example, a sufficiently refined risk-adjusted capitation payment system for insurers must be developed and implemented, as well as a functional description of the basic benefits package. Politically, the introduction of basic insurance largely financed by an income-related premium involves substantial income re-distribution. The reforms are complex. The core element of the market-oriented reforms — the transfer of responsibility for cost containment and efficiency from government to the insurers, providers and insureds — cannot be implemented overnight. Therefore, the reforms must be implemented step by step. But the step-by-step approach involves further complexities. Each step should be as balanced as the entire reform blueprint. The Dutch experience teaches us that this is difficult. There are always political groups or powerful interest groups who will find a particular step disadvantageous and try to block it. A technical obstacle to step-by-step implementation is that new legislation may conflict with legislation that is still in force and that must be removed at the next step.

The Dutch experience also shows that it is difficult to realistically schedule full implementation of radical reforms. The original projected implementation period was four years, whereas a realistic period would have been 10 to 15 years. However, setting a time limit for such a politically sensitive issue as health care financing is even more difficult when a government is in office for only four years. On the other hand, if a realistic time frame had been presented in 1988 it is doubtful that the changes we have seen over the past five years, under pressure of a tight deadline, would have taken place.

No Free Market in Health Care

It should be pointed out that the Dutch proposal is not for a free market in health care. A free market in health care would have effects that most societies consider undesirable. In a free market, most low-income and chronically ill people would not have access to the health care they require. In a free market for health insurance, premiums are based on expected costs, which implies that a premium paid by an 80-year-old is on average tenfold that paid by a 20-year-old, and that a chronically ill person pays many times what a healthy person in the same age group does. Also, the insurer might refuse to cover high-risk cases ("burning houses") or might exclude pre-existing medical conditions from coverage.

The Dutch proposal involves "*regulated* competition."[20] Government regulation will not fade away, but its emphasis will change dramatically. Instead of directly controlling volume, prices, and productive capacity, the government must create the conditions necessary to prevent the undesirable effects of a free market from occurring and to let the market meet social goals with respect to health care. A key goal is access to quality care for everyone. The emphasis of government regulation will therefore be primarily on mandatory health insurance for everyone, on the risk-adjusted capitation payments to insurers, anti-cartel measures, quality control and disclosure of information. Therefore the Dutch reform could be described as "re-regulation" rather than "deregulation."

Preventing Cream Skimming

Another lesson of the Dutch experience concerns the crucial role played by a system of sufficiently refined risk-adjusted capitation payments. In the Netherlands we are now in the midst of a vicious circle. In 1993–94, sickness funds are receiving an age-gender adjusted payment per insured. Because of the inaccuracy of these payments, sickness funds are held responsible for only three percent of the difference between their actual expenses and their predicted expenses based on age and gender. However, as long as government bears responsibility for the remaining 97 percent, the funds have few incentives to improve efficiency. And as long as they do not have those incentives, the government will try to retain its old tools of cost containment. This vicious circle can be broken only if the government finds a viable system of sufficiently refined risk-adjusted capitation payments — which we believe is feasible for non-catastrophic risks such as drugs, hospital care and physician services. However, the practical implementation of such a payment system requires data collection, research and administrative efforts.

Those who are not convinced of the potential solutions to the cream skimming problem may favour the combination of a monopsonistic market for health insurance and a competitive provider market. However, the prevention of cream skimming is relevant not only for a competitive health insurance market. It is also relevant for a competitive provider market, in which competing groups of providers receive an *ex ante* determined capitation payment to provide (or to purchase) a defined set of services to a defined population group, such as the GP fundholders in the UK.[21]

Whether cream skimming will be more or less of a problem in a regulated competitive insurance market than in a competitive provider market remains an open question. On the one hand, providers have more opportunities for cream skimming than insurers do because they probably have better information about the riskiness of their patients and because they can use subtler tools. ("My colleague around the corner is very specialized in treating your disease.") On the other hand, providers may be more reluctant to skim than insurers because of more powerful ethical restraints. Therefore, the question of how to prevent cream skimming in a regulated competitive health care market poses a challenge to all countries that intend to implement market-oriented reforms in health care.

1. A. C. Enthoven, "Consumer Choice Health Plan: A National Health Insurance Proposal Based on Regulated Competition in the Private Sector," *New England Journal of Medicine,* Vol. 298, no. 13 (March 1978), pp. 709–20.

2. Ministry of Welfare, Health and Cultural Affairs, *Verandering verzekerd* [Changes assured], Tweede Kamer, 1987–88, 19945 (27-28), March 1988.

3. F. T. Schut, "Workable Competition in Health Care: Prospects for the Dutch Design," *Social Science and Medicine,* Vol. 35, no. 12 (1992), pp. 1445–55.

4. See Ministry of Welfare, Health and Cultural Affairs, *Verandering verzekerd.*

5. Ministry of Welfare, Health and Cultural Affairs, *Werken aan zorgvernieuwing* [Working on renewing health care], Tweede Kamer, 1989–90, 21545 (2), May 1990.

6. Besides compulsory health insurance, people will be free to buy supplemental health insurance (e.g., for a private room). The premium for this voluntary supplemental insurance will not be regulated or subsidized.

7. E. Elsinga, "Political Decision-Making in Health Care: The Dutch Case," *Health Policy,* Vol. 11, no. 3 (June 1989), pp. 243–55.

8. A. Wagstaff and E. K. A. van Doorslaer, "Equity in the Finance of Health Care: Some International Comparisons," *Journal of Health Economics,* Vol. 11, no. 4 (December 1992), pp. 361–87.

9. See Schut, "Workable Competition in Health Care."

10. In this paper we will consider the terms "insurer" and "third-party purchaser of health care" as synonyms.

11. R. C. J. A. Van Vliet and W. P. M. M. van de Ven, "Towards a Budget Formula for Competing Health Insurers," *Social Science and Medicine,* Vol. 34, no. 9 (1992), pp. 1035–48.

12. For an overview of the strategies that can be pursued by insurers to engage in cream skimming as well as for the measures that government can take to prevent it, see W. P. M. M. van de Ven and

R. C. J. A. Van Vliet, "How Can We Prevent Cream Skimming in a Competitive Health Insurance Market? The Great Challenge for the 90s," in P. Zweifel and H. E. Frech (eds.), *Health Economics Worldwide* (Dordrecht: Kluwer, 1992).

13. Of course, at the *aggregate* level, age, gender and region explain a great deal of the variance in health care expenditures among *groups.* The fewer the groups, the higher the proportion of explained variance. However, with respect to the problem of cream skimming in individual health insurance markets the explained portion of the variance of expenditures at the *individual* level is the relevant criterion.

14. See Van Vliet and van de Ven, "Towards a Budget Formula for Competing Health Insurers."

15. See Ministry of Welfare, Health and Cultural Affairs, *Werken aan zorgvernieuwing.*

16. G. B. Nijhuis, "Handelingen Tweede Kamer," October 4, 1988, ZFW/AWBZ, pp. 7–382; E. Veder-Smith, "Handelingen Eerste Kamer," December 13, 1988, pp. 11–405; D. M. Sluimers, Deputy Director-General, Ministry of Health, interview in INZET, nr. 11, 1988, p. III–V. This false argument was also put forward by the Secretary of State for Health, Hans Simons, in a public debate on the Simons Plan held at Erasmus University, Rotterdam, May 17, 1993.

17. We implicitly make the logical assumption that the weights to be given to each risk factor in the formula will be determined in such a way that the weighted average of the risk factors is the best predictor of the individual's cost the following year. So we exclude the absurd formula in which prior-year costs have weight one and other risk factors have weight zero. Even if prior-year costs were the only risk factor included in the capitation formula, its weight in the best predictive formula would be about 0.2. Such a capitation formula will generally not reduce the insurer's incentive for efficiency.

18. W. P. M. M. van de Ven *et al.,* "Risk-adjusted Capitation Payment: The Achilles Heel of Market-Oriented Health Care Reform," paper presented at the annual meeting of the Association for Health Services Research, San Diego, June 4, 1994.

19. Van de Ven and Van Vliet, "How Can We Prevent Cream Skimming in a Competitive Health Insurance Market?," pp. 23–46.

20. "Regulated competition" is not a contradiction in terms. The opposite of "competition" is "monopoly," while the opposite of "regulation" is "free market."
21. M. Matsaganis and H. Glennerster, "The Threat of Cream Skimming in the Post-Reform NHS," *Journal of Health Economics,* Vol. 13, no. 1 (March 1994), pp. 31–60.

J O S H U A   M .   W I E N E R

M ANAGED C OMPETITION AS F INANCING R EFORM :

A V IEW FROM THE U NITED S TATES

Starting with the endorsement of presidential candidate Bill Clinton in September 1992, the dominant framework for health care reform in the United States has been "managed competition."[1] Although numerous specific proposals have been made, all managed competition schemes depend on private insurance to finance care and price competition among health plans to control costs.[2] Among the proposals, only President Clinton's plan and its descendants involve anything like the "global budgets" found in Canada, Germany and other countries.[3] Thus, President Clinton's plan would create an "internal market" for health care.

American advocates of managed competition contend that this approach has several advantages. It builds on the existing American system, which means that it is less disruptive than other reform proposals. About 70 percent of Americans under age 65 have private health insurance, and price is already an important factor in the (largely employer) choice of health plans.[4] By having price competition take place when insurance is purchased, rather than when health care services are used, managed competition does not ask the sick patient to argue with the doctor about fees or about the necessity of an additional test.[5] Moreover, by depending on markets, it encourages private sector creativity, empowers consumers and allows for personal choice.

In the American context, the greatest political virtue of managed competition is what it is not — namely, it is *not* direct government provision or financing of care. Since it expands private rather than public insurance coverage, managed competition ostensibly relies on private insurance premiums rather than direct taxation.[6] Market driven, its appeal is its contention that it does not depend on regulatory controls, which are perceived to be neither effective nor efficient.

By relying on the creativity and vitality of the private sector, advocates hope to avoid some of the inadequacies of the Canadian and European systems. Although their universal coverage and lower costs are the envy of the US, delivery systems in Canada and Europe seem relatively rigid, with substantially longer hospital stays, less substitution of outpatient for inpatient services, and less use of state-of-the-art technologies.[7]

With its emphasis on making markets work, managed competition clearly fits President Clinton's notion that government should "steer, not row."[8] The thesis of this paper, however, is that this perception is wrong, that managed competition requires a Herculean amount of "rowing." Ironically, although much of the appeal of managed competition is that it avoids direct government financing, fixing the health insurance market so that there is fair and equitable price competition turns out to be complex and to require much government intervention and bureaucracy.

COMPETITION IN THE EXISTING SYSTEM

There is, of course, a great deal of competition among health insurers and providers in the US. Much of this competition is undesirable because it leads to higher costs and the exclusion of some people from health insurance.

Current price competition among private insurers is largely based on risk selection, or "cherry picking," rather than efficiency, effectiveness or quality. Because they are unable to control the price or volume of services, health insurers concentrate instead on screening out high-cost sick or disabled persons as a means of maintaining premiums at competitive levels. Medical underwriting, with its waiting periods, pre-existing condition exclusions and blacklisting of entire industries, is now commonplace, especially for insurance sold to small and medium-sized firms.[9] As a result, the people who need insurance the most are increasingly being kept from obtaining it.

There is less price competition among providers, although it is increasing, primarily through negotiated discounts with managed care organizations. Instead, providers compete to have the latest, most expensive and most esoteric medical equipment. For example, hospitals are rushing to purchase $3-million "gamma knives," which are used for very rare neurosurgery.[10] By some estimates, only six of these high-tech machines are needed for all of the US, yet there are already two in Coral Gables, Florida. There are no federal controls over the purchase of expensive technologies by hospitals and physicians. Some states do have "certificate of need" programmes that require approval for large capital expenditures, but these programmes are widely thought to be ineffective.

As the American health policy debate proceeds, there is a decreasing willingness to take the steps necessary to achieve universal coverage, even though the overwhelming majority of Americans endorse it as an abstract principle.[11] However, price competition without universal coverage likely will have negative effects on access for the uninsured. Providers, especially hospitals, currently supply a substantial amount of free care to the uninsured. Controlling for health status, the uninsured receive half to two thirds the amount of health care that the insured receive.[12] Providers who supply uncompensated care recover their costs by raising the prices charged to the insured population.[13] In competitive environments, where it is hard to shift costs to other payers, providers respond by providing less free care.[14]

WHAT IS "MANAGED COMPETITION?"[15]

Managed competition means different things to different people, but at its core it seeks to change the basis on which health insurers and providers compete. Managed competition schemes organize large numbers of people into geographically based health insurance purchasing cooperatives, or, as the Clinton Administration likes to call them, "health alliances." These cooperatives negotiate with insurers and Health Maintenance Organizations (HMOs) to offer insurance to people in the alliance. Within the purchasing cooperative, individuals have the choice of a great many plans, which vary by price. The large number of persons in the alliance would allow for reduced prices, through lower administrative costs, and for the spreading of risks, and would establish a mechanism through which price competition among plans could take place. To make it clear to employees that certain plans are high cost, employers make the same contribution across all plans; thus, people who choose expensive policies must pay the difference out-of-pocket.

Several mechanisms for the reduction or elimination of risk selection have been proposed. First, there is a standard benefit package that all insurers must offer; thus, some plans will not appear to be less expensive than others for the simple reason that they provide fewer benefits. Second, medical underwriting is eliminated; insurers must accept all applicants, regardless of health status. Premiums are adjusted according to the health care "risk" of enrollees and are based on the cost of all persons enrolled in an insurer's plan rather than on the cost experience of individual firms. Thus, no plan will appear to be less expensive simply because it has healthier people enrolled.

In order to make the market more equitable, there are subsidies for low- and moderate-income persons to help them purchase health insurance and to mitigate the cost-sharing burdens. The goal is to give these persons the financial resources to participate in the market for health insurance.

In the Clinton plan, but not in other managed competition proposals, there are also global budgets in the form of government-imposed limits on the weighted-average insurance premium, rather than limits on hospital spending or physician spending, *per se.*[16] These global budgets are anathema to managed competition purists, and are promoted by the Clinton Administration only as a back-up system if competition should fail to control costs. Said candidate Clinton, "Managed competition, not price controls, will make the budget work and maintain quality."[17]

THE ORGANIZATION AND TECHNOLOGY OF MANAGED COMPETITION

It is extremely difficult to organize the market so that health insurance plans and HMOs compete fairly on price and quality. In at least three areas — risk adjustment, quality measurement and the health alliances — the reach of managed competition is beyond its grasp.

First, under managed competition the insurance premiums will be "risk adjusted." This issue is discussed in detail by van de Ven and Schut and by Hamilton elsewhere in this volume; suffice it to say here that the existing technology is inadequate to the task and that major technological breakthroughs in the near future seem unlikely.[18] Moreover, research-driven risk adjusters may require too much data to be administratively practical on a routine basis. While the standard benefit package, the large number of people in the health alliance and the theoretical ability of everyone to enrol in all plans lessens the likelihood of risk selection, the returns to the insurance companies of "cherry picking" are so large as to make this lack of risk-adjustment technology a significant problem.

Second, insurance plans are supposed to compete on quality as well as price. Thus, managed competition plans generally call for the collection of information on the quality of care provided in each health plan, which will then be made available to consumers. As with risk adjustments, the rhetoric about quality measurement outdistances the technological ability to produce. There is not much consensus on what quality *is,* let alone how to measure it. Efforts to develop "report cards" for HMOs have been fairly primitive.[19] Moreover, while it is possible to gather information on patient satisfaction with each health plan, measuring patient satisfaction is not the same as measuring quality of care. In addition, for many aspects of care it is possible to gather information, but interpreting the data is another matter. For example, a 50-percent Caesarean rate is almost certainly too high, and a five-percent rate is probably too low, but what is the ideal level? Aside from the issue of measurement technology, gathering the data to develop useful information is likely to be a major administrative burden for plans; furthermore, detailed government rules on collection of data will be required.

Third, the organizational centrepiece of managed competition is the large purchasing cooperatives or health alliances. In the Clinton plan, 80 percent of the non-elderly population will purchase its health insurance through these organizations; the other 20 percent, who work for large firms, will receive their insurance through "corporate alliances" run by the individual companies.

Establishing and running a national system of health alliances in a country as large as the US would be a daunting task. To begin with, since no health alliances currently exist, 100 to 150 of these organizations would have to be created in a relatively short period of time. The alliances would have to negotiate with and monitor insurance plans, but the really difficult task would be handling the enrolment of approximately 180 million people.

In order to execute the enrolment process, at least 10 complicated tasks would have to be completed over a three- to four-month period each year: (1) All persons in a geographic area would have to be identified and linked by family. (2) Each family would have to be categorized as to whether they will be served through the regular health alliance or the corporate alliance. (3) Each family unit would have to be categorized according to the income-related subsidy to which it is entitled. (4) Each family unit would have to be assessed for its contribution to the risk adjustment. (5) Each family would have to receive from the health alliance a listing of the available health plans, information (including quality) about each, the premium for each, and an enrolment form. (6) The alliance would have to receive and record the choice of plan, either directly from the family or through employers; families who fail to enrol or who complete the form improperly would have to be contacted. (7) For HMOs or other plans that have limited enrolment capacity, any over-enrolment would have to be assigned to other plans and the family would have to be notified. (8) The list of enrollees, their family status, and their subsidy status would have to be transmitted to the insurance companies. (9) If an individual is working, the size and average wage of the company would have to be determined to assess the firm's eligibility for subsidy. (10) Billions of dollars in payments would have to be received, either from the government or directly from employers, and then dispersed to insurance plans based on their enrolment.

This is a lot to expect, even for an established organization. The risk of administrative breakdown is substantial. Indeed, perhaps the worst nightmare for the patient under a system of managed competition would be to telephone a health alliance at an "800" number and receive only a busy signal, or to get through and find oneself not listed in the computer. The real question is whether 100 to 150 organizations capable of performing these tasks can be created.

Probably no component of managed competition has proved to be more unpopular than the health alliances. They have been incessantly attacked as giant new bureaucracies, with too much regulatory authority and too little accountability to consumers and the public-at-large. Indeed, mandatory participation in the health alliances was one of the first elements of President Clinton's plan to be discarded by Congress.

Despite their political unpopularity and their overwhelming administrative burdens, however, mandatory health alliances covering a large majority of the population would perform critical functions that would otherwise be difficult to carry out — the most important of which is ensuring that everyone has an opportunity to enrol in all of the plans. Without the health alliance as a central marketplace providing plan information to large numbers of people, insurance companies would be able to selectively target and enrol individuals and families.[20]

Compromise measures that reduce the role of the health alliance have their own problems. For example, health alliances could be responsible for much smaller numbers of people — the uninsured, welfare recipients and businesses of fewer than 100 employees. However, this means that enrollees will be disproportionately low-income, making participation undesirable to middle-class employees. Instead of eagerly joining the health alliances because of the vastly greater choices and lower premiums, people will be clamouring to get out. Voluntary rather than mandatory participation would create inherently unstable risk pools, because any individual or employer who can obtain cheaper insurance outside the alliance will do so, leaving only the sicker, more expensive population, which will cause premiums to rise. Finally, having more than one health alliance in a geographic area would be an invitation to engage in inter-alliance competition based on risk selection rather than efficiency.

COST CONTAINMENT

Managed competition differs from many other cost-containment strategies in that it focusses on the macro level of health plans rather than on the micro level of when a provider treats a patient.[21] With the exception that they must offer "community-rated" premiums and the uniform benefit package, and must not medically underwrite, insurance plans and HMOs can do whatever is necessary to control costs. Thus, health plans can reduce use and emphasize use of low-cost providers (such as nurse midwives) instead of high-cost providers (such as obstetricians), substitute outpatient for inpatient services, negotiate lower reimbursement rates and reduce administrative costs. Politically, this means that insurance plans, not the government, will have to make the tough decisions on how to control costs. Federal policy makers will be engaged in "aerial bombing" rather than "hand-to-hand combat" on health care costs.

Managed competition purists depend heavily on changing the tax treatment of health insurance as the hammer for cost containment. Employer contributions toward the cost of health insurance are currently an unlimited tax-deductible expense.[22] In addition, these employer contributions are not counted as income for employees, for either income- or payroll-tax purposes. Managed competition theorists believe that this encourages employees to take their compensation in unduly generous and inefficient health insurance.[23] Therefore, they would limit the tax benefits to the level of the "lowest-cost" or at least "low-cost" health plan, providing the basic benefits only. People wishing to use a more expensive insurer or wishing to buy more comprehensive insurance benefits could do so, but would have to pay income and payroll taxes on any employer contribution beyond the limit, or tax cap. President Clinton's plan has a tax cap, but it is a very weak one and would be phased in over a very long period of time.

A tax cap has several policy virtues. It could raise a substantial amount of revenue, is reasonably progressive in its tax effects, and would provide more incentives for insurers to control costs. Still, it is unclear that by itself a tax cap could do much to reduce the rate of growth in health spending. Moreover, a tax cap would be administratively complex to implement.

Advocates have almost certainly exaggerated the likely cost-containment effect of a tax cap. The direct federal revenue loss attributable to not treating employer contributions for health insurance as income will be about US$75 billion in 1994.[24] Even a tax cap that cut revenue losses by a third (US$25 billion) would not likely provide a very dramatic incentive to control costs, given that overall health spending in 1994 will be about US$1 trillion.

Nor is a tight tax cap politically feasible. Unions strongly oppose it because they have given up wage increases to get generous health benefits and do not want a tax increase for their members. But opposition is broader than that. President Bush had to remove a tax cap from his health reform package to mollify Republicans in the House of Representatives. Regardless of its policy virtues, a tough tax cap is a tax increase and it will be strongly resisted.

Moreover, although simple in theory, a properly crafted tax cap may be unadministerable, at least in a country as large as the US.[25] While it is easy to set a single national cap on the deductibility of health insurance, virtually all managed competition proposals would have the cap determined by the market at the health alliance level. An initial problem is setting the "benchmark plan," which would determine the level of the tax cap. The lowest-cost plan is likely to be an HMO, probably one with limited enrolment capacity and one that may not even serve the entire health alliance area. Alternatively, the tax cap could be set at the level of the lowest-cost plans accounting for some proportion of the eligible population — for example, 30 percent. This approach has the drawback that nobody knows in advance what enrolments will be, but the whole purpose of the tax cap is prospectively to influence enrolment choices.

In addition, to the extent that premiums vary by age or family type, the cap would have to vary with those categories. As White points out, assuming an average of two health alliances per state, two age groups and four family types, there would be 800 tax-deductible premium levels.[26] Conceivably, married couples who both work outside the home and are employed in different alliance areas would be subject to different tax caps. Any corporation that had employees in different alliances would be operating under multiple tax codes. Aaron notes, "Attempts to make these rules work would give new meaning to complexity in tax administration and compliance."[27]

While setting a tax cap has its difficulties, so does enforcing global budgets based on insurance premiums. Global budgets at the premium rather than the provider level have the advantage of allowing health plans to shift expenditures among different categories of service, but they are difficult to run.[28] The central point of a global budget is to make the aggregate sum of all premiums equal a prospectively set, societally determined amount. However, since plans are competing according to price, their premiums, by definition, must differ. The problem is that nobody knows for sure, especially when the system is beginning, how many people will enrol in each plan. Thus, total premiums cannot be known. And if competition is to be effective, market shares among plans must be relatively unstable over time. It seems inevitable that aggregate premiums will not equal the externally determined targets. Within the Clinton plan, concerns about maximizing choice of health plan and efforts to make the health alliances less regulatory weakened the authority of the alliances to limit participation of high-cost plans or otherwise to negotiate price reductions.

MANAGED COMPETITION AND EQUITY

Markets are in general a good way to achieve efficiency, but they are often inequitable. By definition, under managed competition individuals and families must pay enough of the insurance premium that price will be an important factor in their choice of plan. Under the Clinton plan, individuals are responsible for 20 percent of the cost of the weighted-average premium, a sum that is probably US$800 to US$1,200 for a family. The equity problem is that without help poor people will not be able to participate in the health plans that rich people do. While this kind of two-tiered system does not bother most people when it comes to car radios, the idea that people should have inferior access to quality health care simply because they have less money is troublesome to most people in the US.[29] This is true even though the current system treats the poor substantially differently from how it treats the middle and upper classes.

To cope with this problem, all plans for managed competition provide for subsidies for low-income and (in some cases) middle-income persons, for both cost sharing and health insurance premiums. To be fair, it should be noted that subsidies are a requirement in all health reform proposals that rely on private insurance, and that subsidies would be necessary even for government-run programmes if they include more than token levels of cost sharing.

Addressing these equity problems raises at least three issues.

The first is the level of subsidy for the low- and moderate-income population. Under the Clinton plan, the poor are fully subsidized up to the cost of the weighted-average premium. This relatively generous subsidy gives the low-income population an opportunity to purchase plans that a substantial portion of the American people are enrolled in. Obviously, however, they would be unable to participate in the costly plans in which upper-income people could afford to enrol. Other proposals are substantially less generous, subsidizing the poor only up to the cost of the lowest-cost plan or the lowest-cost plan that includes a reasonable number of enrollees. In addition, in order to lessen the economic burden of an employer mandate on small businesses, the Clinton plan and other proposals include substantial subsidies for small, low-wage companies.

Second, providing subsidies to large numbers of people will require enormous administrative effort and expense. Under President Clinton's proposal, people under 150 percent of the federal poverty level will be eligible for subsidies; under other plans, people with even higher income would be eligible. At 150 percent of the federal poverty level, approximately a quarter of the non-elderly American population, 55 million, would be eligible for subsidies, more than four times the recipients of

Aid to Families with Dependent Children, the principal welfare programme.[30] Adding to the complexity, since all the plans call for the amount of subsidy to vary by income, each family's level of income would have to be fairly precisely determined. In addition, small-business subsidies would create perverse incentives for companies to portray themselves as small and low-wage, even when they are not, and would involve another layer of administrative reporting, certification and enforcement.

Third, phasing out the subsidy by income level amounts to an implicit income tax. Combined with other features of the American tax code, including federal and state income taxes, payroll taxes and the earned-income tax credit (an income supplement for low-wage workers), the effective marginal tax rate for relatively low- to moderate-income people would be more than 60 percent in most proposals.[31] That is, for each additional dollar earned, government benefits would be reduced by 60 cents. Obviously, this is a major work disincentive and conflicts with efforts to reduce dependence on welfare. It is possible to reduce these marginal tax rates, but only by increasing the proportion of the population eligible for the subsidy, which means higher costs and the need for even more people to submit to an income determination, or by reducing the subsidy for the very poor, which would be inequitable.

CONCLUSIONS

President Clinton and other proponents of managed competition with global budgets have put forth a variety of plans to radically transform the American health care system. These proposals were not enacted in 1994. This is a result of some general factors in the American health care system and some factors peculiar to managed competition. The core dilemma in the American politics of health care is that all industrialized countries achieve universal coverage and lower costs than the US because in those countries governments play a larger role in health care than government does in the US. But Americans have low regard for their governments and do not want to see them play a more important role.

Managed competition attempts to handle this political problem by retaining private insurers but changing the rules of the game by which they compete. Thus, advocates of managed competition extol the virtues of the market and denounce government regulations. To the surprise of many such advocates, making the market work turns out to be quite complicated, cumbersome, regulatory and bureaucratic. The Clinton Administration added to this complexity by proposing strong global budgets, but it consistently downplayed the importance of these regulatory controls, maintaining that costs actually would be controlled by market forces. Ironically, by accepting the anti-government rhetoric of opponents of more direct government financing of health care, the Administration was unable to respond when its proposal was attacked as relying too much on government regulation. But it is the regulatory approaches of global budgets and rate regulation, not price competition, that have the proven record of controlling costs in health care.[32]

What lessons can Canada and Europe draw from the American effort to design and enact managed competition with a global budget?

First, having multiple health insurance plans compete creates enormous incentives for risk selection, which are not easily solvable with the current technology for risk adjustment. Serious efforts to reduce insurance company-driven risk selection require a complicated administrative structure. Countries like Canada, which have only a single health plan in a geographic area, do not have to worry about risk selection.

Second, if health insurance plans are to have meaningful competition, there must be some factors that differentiate plans fairly. Health systems like those of Canada and most of Europe, which allow free choice of providers and reimburse hospitals and physicians on a uniform fee schedule, do not leave much basis on which health plans could compete other than risk selection.

And, finally, if insurance plans vary substantially in price and if individuals are expected to pay a substantial portion of the cost out-of-pocket, then administratively complicated systems of income-related subsidies are essential as a matter of equity. In Canada and most European countries, this is unnecessary because the funds for the health system are raised on a more or less income-related basis that automatically provides subsidies to low- and moderate-income families. In addition, the low or non-existent levels of cost sharing in other countries means that subsidies are not needed at point-of-service.

In sum, there is no doubt room for the application of market mechanisms to health care in Canada and Europe. However, as other countries explore these competitive approaches, they should be careful not to compromise what they treasure most about their health insurance systems.

1. Bill Clinton, "A Healthy Nation," speech delivered in Rahway, NJ, September 24, 1992.

2. Alain C. Enthoven and Richard Kronick, "A Consumer-Choice Health Plan for the 1990s: Universal Health Insurance in a System Designed to Promote Quality and Economy," *New England Journal of Medicine,* Vol. 320, no. 1 (January 5, 1989), pp. 29–37, and no. 2 (January 12, 1989), pp. 94–101; Paul M. Ellwood, Alain C. Enthoven and Lynn Etheridge, "The Jackson Hole Initiative for a Twenty-First Century American Health Care System," *Health Economics,* Vol. 1, no. 3 (1992), pp. 149–68; and Alain C. Enthoven, "The History and Principles of Managed Competition," *Health Affairs,* Vol. 12 (Supplement 1993), pp. 24–48.

3. Joseph White, *Competing Solutions: American Health Care Proposals and the International Experience* (Washington, DC: The Brookings Institution, forthcoming 1995). For the theoretical rationale for managed competition with global budgets, see Paul Starr and Walter A. Zelman, "Bridge to Compromise: Competition Under a Budget," *Health Affairs,* Vol. 12 (Supplement 1993), pp. 7–23.

4. Employee Benefit Research Institute, "Sources of Health Insurance and Characteristics of the Uninsured: Analysis of the March 1993 Current Population Survey," *Special Report and Issue Brief,* no. 145 (January 1994), table 1, p. 5.

5. According to Alain Enthoven, "Managed competition is price competition, but the price it focuses on is the annual premium for comprehensive health care services, not the price for individual services. There are several reasons for this. First, the annual premium encodes the total annual cost per person. It gives the subscriber an incentive to choose the health plan that minimizes total cost. Second, it is the price that people can understand and respond to most effectively, during the annual enrollment, when they have information, choices, and time for consideration. Third, sick, non-expert patients and their families are in a particularly poor position to make wise decisions about

long lists of individual services they might or might not need. They need to rely on their doctors to advise what services are appropriate and their health plans to get good prices. For economical behaviour to occur, doctors must be motivated to prescribe economically. Managed competition is compatible with selected copayments and deductibles for individual services that can influence patients to do their part in using resources wisely and that are price signals that patients can understand and to which they can respond." Enthoven, "The History and Principles of Managed Competition," pp. 29–30. In addition, available evidence suggests that the price elasticity for health insurance is higher than it is for individual services. For a review, see Michael A. Morrissey, *Price Sensitivity in Health Care: Implications for Health Care Policy* (Washington, DC: National Federation of Independent Businesses Foundation, 1992).

6.   Whether mandatory private insurance premiums are actually taxes is a matter of intense debate. For a discussion, see Congress of the United States, *An Analysis of the Administration's Health Proposal* (Washington, DC: Congressional Budget Office, February 1994).

7.   George J. Schieber, Jean-Pierre Poullier and Leslie M. Greenwald, "US Health Expenditure Performance: An International Comparison and Data Update," *Health Care Financing Review,* Vol. 14, no. 4 (Summer 1992), pp. 1–88; Dale A. Rublee, "Medical Technology in Canada, Germany and the United States," *Health Affairs,* Vol. 8, no. 3 (Fall 1989), pp. 178–81; and William E. Schmidt, "British Health System Fails Cancer Victims, Critics Say," *New York Times,* June 26, 1994, pp. 1, 6.

8.   David Osborne and Ted Gaebler, *Reinventing Government: How the Entrepreneurial Spirit is Transforming the Public Sector* (Reading, Mass.: Addison-Wesley, 1992).

9.   Joshua M. Wiener and Jeannie Engel, *Improving Access to Health Services for Children and Pregnant Women* (Washington, DC: The Brookings Institution, 1991), pp. 36–38.

10.   George Anders, "High-Tech Health: Hospitals Rush to Buy $3 Million Device Few Patients Can Use," *Wall Street Journal,* April 20, 1994, pp. A1, A6.

11.   In a *Washington Post*-ABC News poll, 78 percent of Americans

"strongly" or "somewhat" support "a system providing universal health insurance coverage for all Americans." David S. Broder and Richard Morin, "Poll Finds Public Losing Confidence in Clinton, Economy," *Washington Post,* June 28, 1994, p. 4.

12. Howard E. Freeman *et al.,* "Uninsured Working-Age Adults: Characteristics and Consequences," *Health Services Research,* Vol. 24, no. 6 (February 1990), p. 817; Mark B. Wenneker, Joel S. Weissman and Arnold M. Epstein, "The Association of Payer with Utilization of Cardiac Procedures in Massachusetts," *Journal of the American Medical Association,* Vol. 264, no. 10 (September 12, 1990), pp. 1255–65; and Jack Hadley, Earl P. Steinberg and Judith Feder, "Comparison of Uninsured and Privately Insured Hospital Patients," *Journal of the American Medical Association,* Vol. 265, no. 3 (January 16, 1991), pp. 374–79.

13. Congress of the United States, "Responses to Uncompensated Care and Public-Program Controls on Spending: Do Hospitals Cost Shift?" in *CBO Papers* (Washington, DC: Congressional Budget Office, May 1993).

14. Jonathan Gruber, "The Effect of Price Shopping in Medical Markets: Hospital Responses to PPOs in California," National Bureau of Economic Research, Working Paper no. 4190 (Cambridge, Mass.: NBER, 1992).

15. The description of the Clinton proposal is taken from *H.R. 3600: The Health Security Act,* 101st Congress, 1st Session.

16. The "weighted-average premium" is the average health insurance premium weighted by the enrolment in each health insurance plan. Thus, a plan with 200,000 enrollees would have twice the weight as a plan with 100,000 enrollees.

17. Press release, Clinton/Gore '92 Committee, Little Rock, Arkansas, October 8, 1992.

18. Joseph P. Newhouse, "Patients at Risk: Health Reform and Risk Adjustment," *Health Affairs,* Vol. 13, no. 1 (Spring 1994), pp. 132–46.

19. See, for example, Kaiser Permanente Northern California Region and Andersen Consulting, *1993 Quality Report Card* and *1993 Quality Report Card Supplement.* Arguably, of the 102 measures only about a

third represent outcomes related to care, and eight of these have no benchmarks. See also Linda Oberman, "Grading the Report Cards," *American Medical News,* February 21, 1994, p. 3; "AMA Panel on Guidelines Sorts Good from Misguided," *American Medical News,* January 10, 1994, p. 1; and Ron Winslow, "Health Care Report Cards Are Getting Low Grades from Some Focus Groups," *Wall Street Journal,* May 19, 1994, p. B9.

20. Paul Starr, "Alliance for Progress," *New York Times,* March 6, 1994, p. E15.

21. Although managed competition and global budgets are the centre-pieces of cost containment in President Clinton's proposal, the plan contains a "kitchen sink" approach to cost containment that also includes rate regulation for fee-for-service health plans, coverage of preventive services, modest levels of cost sharing at the point of service, changing the supply of physicians to favour primary care and a weak "tax cap" that would eventually limit the tax deductibility of health insurance.

22. Congress of the United States, *The Tax Treatment of Employment-Based Health Insurance* (Washington, DC: Congressional Budget Office, 1994).

23. Enthoven and Kronick, "A Consumer-Choice Health Plan for the 1990s."

24. Congress of the United States, *The Tax Treatment of Employment-Based Health Insurance.*

25. Henry J. Aaron, "Testimony," Committee on Education and Labour, US House of Representatives, Washington, DC, March 3, 1994; and White, *Competing Solutions.*

26. White, *Competing Solutions.*

27. Aaron, "Testimony."

28. Joseph White, "Managing the Right Premium," *Journal of Health Politics, Policy and Law,* Vol. 19, no. 1 (Spring 1994), pp. 255–59.

29. Not to everyone, however. For a strong defence of two-tiered health systems, see H. Tristram Engelhardt, Jr., "Why a Two-Tier System of Health Care Delivery is Morally Unavoidable," in Martin A. Strosberg *et al.* (eds.), *Rationing America's Medical Care: The Oregon Plan and Beyond* (Washington, DC: The Brookings Institution, 1992), pp. 196–207.

30. Employee Benefit Research Institute, "Sources of Health Insurance and Characteristics of the Uninsured: Analysis of the March 1993 Current Population Survey," table 14, p. 33; and US Bureau of the Census, *Statistical Abstract of the United States, 1993* (Washington, DC: US Government Printing Office, 1993), table 604, p. 381.
31. Aaron, "Testimony."
32. White, *Competing Solutions.*

JOSEPH WHITE

MANAGING HEALTH CARE COSTS

IN THE UNITED STATES

The American debate on health care cost control starts from a place very different from that of the debate in Canada or any other country represented in this volume. In those countries the question is how to control costs while continuing to guarantee some decent standard of health care to all members of society;[1] a system in which costs are to be controlled is taken for granted, even if the level of control is contentious. In the United States the issue is not only whether and how to control costs and extend coverage; it is also whether to have a system in which one could plausibly discuss cost control.

The US has many advocates of markets but not so many supporters of internal markets. The word "internal" implies a market that operates within an envelope of resource constraint. In normal markets — say, for automobiles or stereo equipment — developments within that market can cause more resources to flow into it. If someone invents a great new sound system, people may buy more stereo equipment. The idea of an internal market implies that market mechanisms allocate resources among participants in a given activity, but that the total amount of resources in that market is not, in fact, allowed to be shaped by the dynamic events within the market. Publicity for a new diagnostic test, for example, should cause re-allocation of resources only from other medical services, and not from spending for new buses or video games or baseball players.

From the standpoint of Canada or Britain or Sweden or the Netherlands, or virtually anywhere else, discussions about an internal market would centre on the creation of some process of allocation by bidding and exchange within the envelope of existing financial arrangements.[2] In the US there is no envelope. There are many proposals for "market-based" reform, but most of these — including the original Jackson Hole version of managed competition — cannot be defined as an "internal market," because they allow no bounds. The only proposal that qualifies is the Clinton Administration plan: "managed competition with a global budget."

The US, therefore, while it has a great deal of experience with so-called market mechanisms, has no experience whatsoever with internal market reforms, properly defined. The meaning of such reforms in the US is entirely different from its meaning in other countries — particularly the United Kingdom. Whatever one may think of so-called competition, how it will work when brought into an American system that has never had much of a resource constraint has to differ greatly from how it will work when interjected into a British world that has been under immense external constraint for decades.

The closest American equivalent to internal market theories — managed competition — presumes that health care costs can be reduced, with acceptable effects on quality, when delivery is managed by plans that must compete for patronage. This is the same presumption that is found in the Dutch reforms, and it is a stronger version of the GP fund-holder system in the UK. Americans do have more experience than anyone else with the basic issue in this idea: whether and how plans of some sort can manage care.

In the companion paper in this section, Joshua Wiener discusses the issues raised by the concept of competition within managed competition. These are issues, such as risk selection, that other countries also must address if they pursue internal market reforms. This paper will consider the problems and prospects of management. It will offer evidence from experience of American managed care, and conclude by discussing the relevance of the American experience for other countries.

One point must be made at the outset. In other countries the notion of an internal market may involve individual providers competing for part of the business available within what was once a system of direct health care delivery, as with the hospital trusts in the UK. The concept of managed care in the US involves a combination of the insurance and care-giving functions. Whether it is for-profit or not-for-profit, an organization competes for business as an insurer, promising to provide care that it then will "manage." The manager offers a full range of health care services. Independent providers may compete for business from the insurer/managers.

TYPES OF MANAGED CARE

There are three main forms of managed care in the US.

The form easiest to create can be called *third-party management.* An insurer contracts with various care-givers to provide care to its beneficiaries. The insurer pays according to a fee schedule, and regulates decisions according to a wide variety of utilization rules such as review of bills for compliance and pre-clearance of procedures.

Utilization review of some sort exists in many systems. In the American context, however, each payer has its own system. In general, care-givers contract with a variety of such payers, each with different rules and different fees. Each payer is only part of the business, and the payers all have different requirements. Administration in the US requires more time and money than it does in any other country, because there are more (different) rules and less prospect for informal, lasting accommodations. Rules regarding treatment are enforced over the telephone by nurses who do not see the patient. In theory, treatments are not rejected without a physician reviewer's say-so; in practice, the hassle factor of appealing from the nurse up the chain to the physician reviewer can be enough to cause a busy care-giver to give up or to negotiate a compromise with the nurse reviewer.[3]

The second form of managed care is the *traditional HMO:* the group- or staff-model Health Maintenance Organization beloved by health policy analysts. In the HMO ideal form, a group of physicians practise together, develop a conservative practice culture, and provide quality, integrated care. If a person needs extraordinary care, the physicians consult with each other and, following their professional norms, agree to provide it.

The physicians in the group serve only patients who contract with the group, and patients visit only the doctors within the group (save for the rare need for outside consultation). The HMO may even own its own hospital. The physicians therefore deal with only one set of rules, and the HMO can develop the kinds of informal social structures that make good organizations work.

I call the third form of managed care the *risk-bearing gatekeeper* model. A primary care physician is given responsibility for both the care and the expense of each patient. There may still be some utilization review, but restrictions in use are made less by outside review than by the primary physician's ensuring that costs remain within limits. If they are higher, the physician is subject to some form of economic sanction; if lower, the physician might receive a bonus (likely nominal).[4]

LOGICS OF MANAGEMENT

Third-party management presumes that rules for treatment can be created, and that outsiders can judge which rules apply to which cases and whether deviations are appropriate. If treatments must be approved in advance, then the condition must allow delay. If they are reviewed in retrospect, the provider must have a reasonable chance of anticipating the result. Review of many elective surgical procedures comes close to meeting the requirements, and reductions in hospital admissions are the greatest evidence of success of this approach.

Everybody, everywhere, wants to find better treatment guidelines, but American reformers — and probably many others — vastly overstate the prospects for inventing them. If guidelines can be found, and if they save money, nobody is coerced and everybody is happier. But there are great obstacles to both developing and implementing such guidelines, and they make least sense in the context of competing managed-care plans.

First, for physicians to accept them, the standards must be authoritative. The most legitimate authority is the profession or specialty itself. It may develop guidelines with government approval, or it may approve guidelines developed by the government; but proprietary standards developed within one plan can never have that authority, and non-proprietary standards cannot create competitive advantage. Second, in the American context providers are subject to a second form of review, the malpractice suit. If a standard were accepted by specialty societies, then following it might be a defence; if it is just the insurer's rule, it has no standing in court.

A variation of detailed review is *profiling:* rather than review each decision, a regulator reviews the pattern of the practice of a physician or other provider. Profiling is a much less invasive form of detailed review, and if it serves to improve a physician's practice, through either education or counselling, it could be useful in the long run. But profiling and direct review face similar problems in a context of competing payers. Each payer needs its own reviewers, so if doctors are dealing with multiple payers there will be many more reviewers. That means that the reviewers usually will be nurses or clerks, not the "control doctors" common in systems where the payers cooperate, such as Germany and France. Doctors are not oriented to listening to nurses. Furthermore, the competing plans all have limited, non-random samples of the work of a given provider; they are therefore likely to misapprehend the practice of a physician and to create an issue where none should exist.

In short, the case for detailed review, which is weak to begin with, is weaker within a system of multiple payers for any one provider than within a single-payer system or one in which payers join forces to regulate providers.

Traditional HMOs avoid most of these problems. They see all of a given physician's practice and review can be mainly collegial. Still, they can reduce utilization only to the extent that they are able to obtain agreement on more conservative practice norms. If a given test or treatment is popular outside, it is hard to resist inside.

Traditional HMOs have other problems. In the American context they tend to have lower and less cost sharing — perhaps a low flat fee per visit and little else. That is partly a matter of marketing but also partly a matter of management: more extensive cost sharing requires more detailed billing, and that creates its own burdens. Yet the likely consequence is to marginally raise costs.[5]

Perhaps a greater problem is the lumpiness of the traditional HMO model. Care-givers build a culture and observe each other by working together in clinics. But this means that HMOs are constrained by their physical plant. As membership grows, services can be constrained to unpopular levels; if new facilities are built, for a while membership will be too low for capacity. Other systems do not have this problem because capital costs are borne by the contracting providers and spread among payers.

Further, the best way to build a practice culture is through recruitment. Even an organization that is good at socialization may depend on recruitment. The US Marines do a lot to build a culture, but it works because people who are unlikely to fit in do not join (or leave quickly!). Inherently, then, systems that rely on building a practice culture cannot be quickly or easily expanded. There may be more physicians who would thrive in those cultures than are currently in them, but it is unlikely that a whole system of competing Kaisers could function like a Kaiser. Selection requires selectivity. One may also try to change the culture of physicians as a whole, but that would be a matter of managing medical education, not of managing care.

Risk-bearing gatekeeper systems are in essence attempts to select providers with more conservative practice styles without the organizational restrictions of creating a traditional HMO. They therefore do not have the same capacity problems. In theory, physicians will learn from the market that they must adjust their behaviours in order to satisfy the insurers who control the supply of patients.

In the extreme, insurers would not even have to worry about treatment appropriateness: they would set financial standards, and how these were met would be the problem of the primary care provider. The risk is to quality. Insurers claim that they choose gatekeepers on the basis of cost and quality of care. But physicians may be right in insisting that cost matters far more than results — for the simple reason that few good outcome measures exist. Insurers do use surrogates for quality such as board certification, and they may carry out surveys of patient satisfaction, but quality measures are extremely rudimentary.[6] Unlike the traditional HMO, the gatekeeper model provides little or no collegial review to help the primary care physician make hard choices. It normally limits in size the set of doctors to whom referrals can be made, yet it does not create the set of relationships that helps doctors assess each other's work.

Unless the primary physician is part of a large group, or part of a small group that relates to a very small number of payers, the model also puts the gatekeeper at risk of suffering the effects of random variation in the needs of patients.

Other systems have tried to save by putting physicians at risk for the costs of their prescribing. Yet these risks remain quite limited. In Britain, GP fundholders are at risk for only about 15 percent of hospitalization costs, and fundholding practices combine the total lists of roughly three GPs.[7] Prescribing physicians in Germany have now been put at financial risk if their total pharmaceutical costs exceed targets, but that is still only a portion of the costs produced by a physician's ordering pen, and one that is relatively easy to control.

Putting a physician at financial risk if an extra two or three out of a few hundred patients has severe illness is a different proposition. A sole practitioner who deals with five insurers becomes, in essence, proprietor of five small beneficiary groups — and can get caught in the same ways in which those groups themselves get hurt by random variation in the current American system. Worse, a physician who is particularly good at treating expensive diseases could be punished for attracting such patients.

COSTS

The US does not quite provide an experiment in the effects of these various systems. There is no coherent database on either costs or, of course, outcomes. Nor is there agreement on a classification scheme. And a degree of third-party managed care is now the norm. One cannot compare these approaches to entirely unmanaged systems because the latter barely exist in the US any more. Differences in the risk profiles of the membership of various plans further inhibits comparison.

Estimates do nevertheless exist. The most important summary was issued in March 1994 by the Congressional Budget Office (CBO).[8] The CBO estimates determine how budget process rules are applied to the deliberations of Congress, so they greatly affect the prospects of each bill. They are based on literature reviews, including some unpublished material.

CBO estimates that a good utilization review system — as compared to none — can save about 3.7 percent of costs.[9] It sees larger savings from HMOs — about nine percent for the best versions, compared to the "typical fee-for-service plan."[10] CBO argues that there are two "effective" forms of HMO: the group or staff model, and an "effective" form of Independent Practice Association (IPA). The most effective forms of IPA are those that "select cost-conscious providers, maintain an effective network for information and control, place providers at financial risk, and generate a substantial portion of each provider's patient load."[11] In other words, CBO's effective IPAs are those that most resemble the gatekeeper model.

These approaches already exist to some extent, and about 30 percent of the nation is so sparsely populated that the HMO model cannot be implemented.[12] CBO therefore estimates the savings that would be made if 70 percent of the population were in effective HMOs and the rest were in effective utilization review systems, and concludes that total savings, relative to the *status quo*, would be about 5.7 percent of what it calls "potentially manageable personal health care expenditures." Relative to the part of the system with least management, Medicare, savings would be seven percent; relative to total national health expenditures, savings would fall to four percent.[13]

These are not exactly promising numbers. In contrast, the Canadian health care system, the second most expensive in the world, had costs in 1991 — before the current severe squeeze in Canada — 25 percent lower than the US system.[14]

OTHER EFFECTS

Managed care greatly affects physicians. Insurers that create limited networks thereby interfere with professional relationships among providers. All models depend on physicians to pay attention to costs and utilization, but the risk-bearing model does so in a particularly nasty way — by punishing physicians who have a sicker than average patient load. Third-party managed care bureaucratizes medicine, requiring extensive non-collegial consultation.

One interesting question is how the pain of these constraints compares to the pain of other cost-control methods. Many American doctors hate managed care — but that does not mean they would prefer alternatives.

American managed care has had the virtues of its weakness. Since it does not work very well, it has not constrained the incomes of physicians. American physicians, unlike those of virtually every other industrialized country, have seen their incomes rise, relative to those of the rest of society, most years over the past decade.[15]

If the movement to managed care were to suddenly yield real cost control, however, the new system would have the evils of its strengths. Managed care works, when it works at all, through payers developing limited lists of providers. They must be able to "de-list" hospitals and doctors on economic grounds. Those grounds may be not that a provider is much more expensive than the average, but that the plan wants to reduce its administrative costs by having more patients per doctor. The agenda of cost control through managed care is to give the insurer the power to manage the providers. From the standpoint of physicians and hospitals this can be a matter not only of independence but of survival, as cost control can mean denying business to some.

A system that controls costs far more by constraining capacity, such as Canada's, creates other problems. Instead of dealing with insurers, physicians must negotiate with colleagues or hospital managers for allocation of beds or operating facilities. While this may be a better way of making decisions, it can be just as stressful for the doctors: many people are more comfortable with impersonal than with personal conflict.

Constrained capacity is not a violation of professional *status:* nonprofessionals do not interfere so much with treatment decisions. However, it remains a serious restriction on one's ability to practise medicine as one's professional training advises — especially in a country like Canada, whose professionals receive essentially the same training as their US counterparts.

Yet limits on payments through fee schedules and facility budgets, and limits on capacity increases, are less disruptive and cause lower risk to both provider and patient than will occur if American managed care suddenly becomes more successful. For the savings they generate, these standard international methods violate professionalism less — and since administration costs are lower they also leave more income for doctors.

The most defensible forms of care management, such as profiling of physician practice patterns, make far more sense as part of a unified system, in which physicians basically review each other and in which all of a given practice is included in the profile, than within a system in which a doctor's practice is divided among separate, managing payers.

The more effective forms of managed care depend on restricted choice of provider. Advocates promise that patients stand to gain because the systems will allow for improved measurement of performance and satisfaction, so that patient choice, though limited, will be better informed. We know, however, that any measurement system will be flawed. We also know that people have their own standards for choosing physicians, such as what they hear from friends or their own experience with a given doctor. There is little appeal in choosing among a limited set of plans according to rating systems devised by experts — and likely criticized extensively by the losers — when the alternative is choosing the doctor recommended by friends.

Managed care, therefore, is more popular with American policy wonks than with the general public. That does not mean that people refuse to participate. People take what they can get, just as they buy whatever cars are on the market. If change is slow enough, they will accommodate themselves. But the charge that choice will be restricted has been a powerful weapon in the American policy debate, even though it has been aimed in the wrong direction. Reformers in other countries have to ask themselves why their publics would accept the restrictions necessary to effectively manage care in competing plans.

CREATING AN ENVELOPE

There are some obvious reasons why competing managed care has not controlled costs in the US as effectively as have systems of regulation in other countries.

1. To the extent that any system saves from bargaining for lower fees, the payers will do better when they have more concentrated power, as in any single-payer or all-payer cartel system, than when the payers compete with each other, as they do in the US.

2. It is easier to restrain costs by not having capacity than by trying to stop people from using capacity that is already there.

3. To the extent that cost control relies on cooperation from professionals, it works better through market-wide negotiations on costs and incomes than through the efforts of separate plans to manage treatments.

4. If managed care means adapting utilization to resource constraints within an organization, other countries have much more successful managed care in the hospital sector, which is more tightly constrained and managed.

5. Systems that adjust prices to volume, of which the German physician payment system is the most stringent, can control costs without directly limiting utilization — though we have no more idea how that affects German quality of care than we have about the effects of American utilization constraints.

Nevertheless, American advocates of managed care claim that it would work better under different circumstances. The right wing emphasizes greater price constraints, such as lower subsidies through the tax system for purchase of insurance. The left wing emphasizes greater budget constraints, such as capping the average premiums within the system.

The budget constraint argument is more germane here — and more plausible. A budget constraint suggests some method for limiting premiums. It involves two issues: First, how will controlling the price of insurance limit the costs of care? And second, how might the premiums be controlled?

Premium limits should cause insurers to behave differently. At present they base their own targets on experience, and fear that stringent cost control will cost them both in customers and in affiliations with providers. Price competition is based on guesses about what rivals can achieve as well as each player's own ability to control costs. Nobody is very good at cost control, everybody knows that, so costs keep rising.

Given premium limits, insurers would have no choice but to try to make costs fit the limits. The difficulty is the kind of medical care system that would result. Clinton Administration optimists believed group- and staff-model HMOs would quickly take over the market in response to constraints. But the capital and recruitment requirements of the model —never mind its lack of popularity — ensure that it could not grow so quickly. Caps are far more likely to result in intensified versions of utilization review and holding gatekeepers to lower cost targets. Payers would also try to negotiate lower fees. But, as noted above, that works better within a system of overall fee-setting than through competition.[16]

Even if the insurers could meet the savings targets, enforcement of a premium cap poses substantial problems. Any spending standard for the services guaranteed all citizens must be set by the primary budget-holder — a province in Canada, likely the federal government in the US. It must be related to the system's income, and accommodate regional variations.

A system based on local general revenue or percentage of income contributions automatically raises money in relation to local levels of incomes and input costs (which track incomes). If the standard is a premium, it may be adjusted for regional variations in levels of incomes and input costs. American proposals made this process much more complicated by relying on fixed-dollar premiums, which therefore had to be adjusted by a national board to accommodate regional differences. That not only provoked charges of "big bureaucracy," but would have created serious political conflict over the calculations.

However a local target is set, reformers have to determine how to translate that into the premiums of competing plans. The government could require that all plans charge the same prices, but allow variation on other dimensions, such as cost sharing, supplemental benefits or the list of providers. The government could claim it was encouraging innovation and some consumer choice of benefits or form of benefits, while maintaining a basic guarantee (though rather more variable than before). That is certainly the logic of the British GP fundholder reforms. Enforcing the overall target, then, is not much a problem — unless one worries about risk adjustments.

But American reformers want price competition among plans. That, in turn, requires methods to ensure that the average of the premiums of all plans weighted by their enrolment, which in the Clinton plan was called the *weighted-average premium,* meets the target.

In some versions of managed competition, plans are allowed to set whatever premiums they choose. The central purchasing group, or alliance, is merely a *price-taker,* forwarding the price list to citizens who then choose among plans. A pure price-taker system cannot enforce targets.

The obvious alternative is to allow managers of the alliance to negotiate with each plan, and attempt to contract for a distribution of prices that will lead to the right weighted average of enrolments. The alliance then must be able to refuse to offer a given plan without agreement on a price. Then the alliance is a *price-maker.*

The most widely cited example of managed competition saving money, the California Public Employees Retirement System, or CalPERS, is a clear example of the power of a price-maker. CalPERS represents so large a part of its insurers' businesses that they dare not lose it. For years CalPERS allowed competition to work without "interference." But in 1992, influenced by a state budget crisis, CalPERS managers got tough. In 1992, they held the average premium increase to 6.1 percent, compared to an 8.6-percent average in the state. In 1993, CalPERS restrained the average increase to 1.4 percent, and demanded premium rollbacks in its initial bargaining position for 1994.[17] While some of the savings were associated with a new co-payment structure that reduced payments for the Kaiser health plans, clearly the market power of CalPERS made a difference.

Yet the major "managed competition" bills in Congress, including Clinton's, did not allow alliances to play this price-making role. The objections to alliances as price-makers (or anything else) were never articulated in an intellectually coherent manner, yet two reasons for protest are evident. First, a price-making alliance is not engaged in a "competitive" process as it is usually understood. It is using pure market power — and that power would be even greater if the alliance represented 70 or 80 percent of the market. Second, it puts a remarkable amount of power in the hands of whoever runs the alliance.

Typically for the US, the Administration instead proposed an extremely complex, formula-based, "Look, Ma, no hands" process. Each plan would make a "bid" of the premium it wanted and the National Health Board would automatically reduce excessive bids. I have analyzed the perversities of the particular proposal elsewhere.[18] For our purposes the point is that neither the Clinton Administration nor anyone else has identified a good way in which to enforce a target average premium.

There is an answer, but not in the terms that the American debate has defined. A regulator can set the *maximum premium* and then allow competition among plans in which plans might charge less than the maximum. In this context, the maximum would apply to fee-for-service care with the country's standard set of benefits and cost sharing. Other plans could offer a combination of lower prices, more benefits and/or lower cost sharing. Competition to manage care might then allow somewhat more value for the money, and slightly lower costs, than direct regulation.

But that approach is possible only if the government admits that it is going to control the cost of fee-for-service medicine through regulation. The Clinton Administration was willing to regulate, but unwilling to defend that choice.

IMPLICATIONS

I have argued that managed care on the American model cannot improve on the methods of cost control that other countries have implemented. The US would do better to adapt those other methods first, and achieve what it can that way.

Policy makers in Canada and overseas nevertheless are attracted to American notions of management and competition. The simplest explanation is that they have accomplished what they can with their methods, and now seek new ones. The agenda of managed care also links up, at least in theory, with a series of other agendas, such as emphasis on preventive medicine and integrated service provision, or on decentralization. The notion of a system of clinics in which physicians and other health professionals coordinate care for the whole person should be familiar to many Canadians, especially Quebecers.

Another attraction is that other countries take their control of fee-for-service costs for granted. Doing better than the US is not seen as an accomplishment; resisting the relentless demographic pressures to spend more of the national wealth on health care is a pressing concern, whether the share is eight or nine or 10 percent of GDP. From any given level of fees and incomes, greater "efficiency" of integrated care may seem a more politically viable approach to cost control than intensification of existing methods. The fact that the US has not reduced its fee-for-service costs to such a low level is not seen as relevant elsewhere.

Most of all, both in the US and abroad the notion of cost control by integrated networks of some sort offers a form of blame avoidance: the government sets a target but the plans are responsible for the consequences of hitting that target.[19] For governments fatigued by conflict with the medical profession and other providers, the prospect of cost control in this new form — wrapped in the rhetoric of integration and wellness — must be attractive.

But so long as patients are guaranteed free choice of provider, with few financial incentives to accept limits, they are not very willing to affiliate with such plans. That creates an ironic situation: the US is likely to create a world of competing integrated plans not because it is more advanced, but because it is more backward.

Patients will accept restricted choice of provider only if coverage with wider choice has some other disadvantage. Restricted-choice plans might have more benefits or lower cost sharing or lower prices. But that is possible only if the basic system is missing some desirable benefits, has cost sharing and/or charges premiums. That is the norm in the US.

An "internal market" of any sort presumes that existing arrangements are in some way inadequate. Without inadequacies — under-supply of services or price constraints that families wish to avoid — there is no basis for competition.

In his companion paper, Joshua Wiener discusses the difficulties of implementing any system of cross-subsidy within a format of competing plans. The discussion of risk selection in other chapters presents another difficulty in implementing a system of competing managed care.

But the most evident political difficulty in a country like Canada is a more fundamental one. Management of care by integrated plans offers governments a way in which to avoid blame for particular savings. But implementing such a plan would explicitly limit choice of physician — something neither voters nor physicians are likely to appreciate. In a country where there is hardly any cost sharing and where insurance is financed basically from general revenues, integrated plans can offer no price advantages. They could offer superior quality only if the quality of fee-for-service medicine were widely believed to be poor. Plans could offer more generous benefits, but that would not reduce the burdens on public budgets.

From south of the border at least, the Canadian system does not yet seem to have the failings needed to convince voters to accept the restrictions of managed care.

1. The guarantee does not necessarily extend to illegal immigrants, nor to persons who refuse to fulfil their obligations to contribute to the system.

2. In the Netherlands, reform is meant to change the financing arrangements but still seems designed to maintain substantial constraints on the resources available. For an account of this rather unsettled situation, see Wynand P.M.M. van de Ven and Frederik T. Schut, "The Dutch Experience with Internal Markets," pp. 95-117 in this volume.

3. Institute of Medicine, Committee on Utilization Management by Third Parties, Bradford H. Gray and Marilyn J. Field (eds.), *Controlling Costs and Changing Patient Care? The Role of Utilization Management* (Washington, DC: National Academy Press, 1989).

4. See David S. Hilzenrath, "In Managed Care, Some Doctors Trip on Bottom Line," *Washington Post,* August 8, 1994, p. A1, for examples of the process.

5. I share Robert Evans' judgement that the main effect of cost sharing is the shifting of costs to the insured. But on balance I am more comfortable saying overall cost reductions are very small than saying they do not exist. For a good review see Jeff Richardson, "The Effects of Consumer Co-payments in Medical Care," Background Paper no. 5, Commonwealth of Australia, National Health Strategy, June 1991.

6. Kaiser Permanente in northern California has developed a report card with some appropriate outcome measures, but it is, of course, a group-model HMO, and the report card is still quite limited. See note 19 in Joshua Wiener's accompanying paper in this volume.

7. See the discussion of fundholding in Howard Glennerster *et al.,* "GP Fundholding: Wild Card or Winning Hand?" in R. Robinson and J. Le Grand (eds.), *Evaluating the NHS Reforms* (London: King's Fund Institute, 1994).

8. Congress of the United States, Congressional Budget Office, *CBO Memorandum,* "Effects of Managed Care: An Update" (March 1994).

9. 4.4 percent of health care costs, of which "about 83 percent of the sav-

ings...remained after allowing for the offsetting increase in administrative costs," Congress of the United States, Congressional Budget Office, *CBO Memorandum,* p. 8.

10. Congress of the United States, Congressional Budget Office, *CBO Memorandum,* p. 21.

11. Congress of the United States, Congressional Budget Office, *CBO Memorandum,* p. 21.

12. R. Kronick *et al.,* "The Marketplace in Health Care Reform," *New England Journal of Medicine,* Vol. 328, no. 2 (January 14, 1993).

13. Kronick *et al.,* "The Marketplace in Health Care Reform," tables 5 and 6, pp. 25–26.

14. In 1991, according to the OECD/CREDES 1993 database, Canada spent 10 percent of GDP on health care and the US spent 13.4 percent.

15. Author's calculations from data in American Medical Association Center for Health Policy Research, *Socio-economic Characteristics of Medical Practice, 1992* (Chicago: American Medical Association, 1992), p. 134; income figures from *Economic Report of the President, 1993;* and Mike Mitka, "Doctor Pay Up 6.5 Percent in 1992; Specialists Benefit Most," *American Medical News,* January 10, 1994, p. 1.

16. The Clinton plan included such measures as a "back-up." The House Ways and Means Committee reform plans included a system with cost controls of this sort as an alternative to the world of competition.

17. United States General Accounting Office, *Health Insurance: California Public Employees' Alliance Has Reduced Recent Premium Growth* (November 1993: GAO/HRD-94-40); also see "CalPERS Tells 18 Health Care Providers It Expects a Five Percent Rollback in Premiums," *Wall Street Journal,* October 14, 1993.

18. For more detail see Joseph White, "Managing the Right Premium," *Journal of Health Politics, Policy and Law,* Vol. 19, no. 1 (Spring 1994), pp. 255–59.

19. R. Kent Weaver, "The Politics of Blame Avoidance," *Journal of Public Policy,* Vol. 6 (1986), pp. 371–98; and Joseph White, "Markets, Budgets, and Health Care Cost Control," *Health Affairs,* Vol. 12, no. 3 (Fall 1993), pp. 44–57.

V I V I A N   H A M I L T O N

RISK SELECTION:

A MAJOR ISSUE IN INTERNAL MARKETS

A DEFINITION OF RISK SELECTION

An internal market for health care relies on efficient competition amongst insurers. These insurers may be third-party payers who reimburse patients or health care providers for expenses incurred, or they may be actively engaged in the provision of both insurance and health care, as Health Maintenance Organizations (HMOs) are in the United States.

Regardless of the organizational form insurers take, policy makers and researchers are concerned with their potential for risk selection in internal markets. Risk selection, also known as "cream skimming," refers to insurers attracting preferred (i.e., low-cost) patients. These preferred risks are insurees for whom the risk-adjusted payment or premium received from the government or the insurer is far above the expected cost level.[1] One of the most serious consequences of risk selection is reduced access to good health care for the chronically ill, since they can be expected to be much more costly than a typical insuree. In addition, efficient insurers, who are willing to enrol both "good" and "bad" risks and contain costs through better management, may be driven out of the health care market by inefficient insurers, who maintain lower costs through risk selection.

Risk selection arises partly as a result of regulation (rather than competition) and partly from a lack of "complete" markets. In a perfectly competitive market, insurers would obtain full premium differentiation for bad *versus* good risks, since those customers who are expected to be quite expensive would simply be charged higher rates.[2] However, given that many health conditions are exogenous ("acts of God") rather than self-inflicted, and that poor health is correlated with lower income, society's preference for equity precludes us from demanding that bad risks bear the full cost of their conditions. Thus, governments have intervened as third-party payers to cover insurance costs. It is this regulatory role of government — in making legal decisions on the structure and classes of the insurance market — that raises the problem of risk selection.

Risk selection may also arise when employers negotiate with third-party payers to purchase HMO-type (per capita) insurance for their employees. In such cases, it is difficult to account for all possible contingencies in the resulting contract, so that rate negotiations lead to payments that do not fully cover the costs of bad risks. Third-party payers will thus attempt to avoid these surplus costs through risk selection.

The concept of risk selection should be distinguished from that of adverse selection. Risk selection is "insurer initiated," and arises when the insurer is better able to predict the cost of certain patient groups than the (risk adjusted) capitation formula. On the other hand, adverse selection is "insuree initiated" (though not always actively), and arises when the insurer is unable to distinguish between good and bad risks. For example, the existing literature which finds that patients enrolling in HMOs have lower health care costs than comparable patients who remain in fee-for-service programmes is not in itself evidence of risk selection by the HMO.[3] The HMO may have *inadvertently* designed a programme that appeals more to good risks. Thus, lower reported health care costs for one insurer *versus* another is a necessary, but not sufficient, condition for evidence of risk selection.

How Does Risk Selection Arise?

To understand how risk selection arises, one need only note that year-to-year medical expenditures vary in a systematic (and observable) manner across different patient groups. For example, young adults generally incur lower costs than the elderly. Due to the availability of increasing amounts of administrative data on health service use in several developed countries, these patient-specific variations are now readily observable by insurers, government regulators, and health care providers.

The observable sources of variation include: (a) sociodemographic characteristics such as age, gender, income, education, and region of residence; (b) level of disability or functional status as measured by competence with activities of daily living (ADLs), or degree of infirmity; (c) chronic conditions such as diabetes, rheumatism, or hypertension; (d) self-rated health; and (e) prior use.[4]

Nevertheless, if risk-adjusted premiums reflect predicted variations in the cost of care for only *some* of these characteristics — just the sociodemographic characteristics, for example — then insurers will use the remaining observables that they can accurately measure to select good (relatively inexpensive) *versus* bad (relatively expensive) risks to enrol in their programmes.

Information on many of these variables is obtainable at the time of enrolment in an insurance programme, particularly if patients are required to undergo a physical examination. Information on other variables, such as income, education, and self-rated health, may be more difficult for the insurer to obtain. Insurers are not legally entitled to ask for this information and verifying patients' self-reports on these data could be costly.

FORMS OF RISK SELECTION

Risk selection can take several forms, many of them quite subtle. For instance, insurers can attempt to attract relatively healthy families by offering extensive maternity benefits and special insurance for sporting accidents. Insurers can also contract with many paediatricians and obstetricians while offering their insurees less access to specialists who care for the chronically ill, such as oncologists, cardiologists, and diabetes specialists. They may engage in direct advertising and marketing in markets dominated by healthy individuals, such as sports enthusiast magazines and television shows.

Unethical practices by insurance companies have been rumoured to occur in the US: at a community dance for the elderly sponsored by an insurance company, for example, only those seniors seen on the dance floor are approached by insurance agents and offered policies; or an insurance company may locate its offices on the second floor of an office building that has no elevator. If an insurer finds that certain persons with poor risks have enrolled, it may try to make these patients wait longer for appointments and sit longer in doctors' waiting rooms. Or the insurer may simply refuse to cover services that are required predominantly by poor risks.

THE POTENTIAL FOR RISK SELECTION IN INTERNAL MARKETS

Several researchers have noted the potential for risk selection in current and proposed internal market systems. Van Vliet and van de Ven have observed that the capitation (i.e., insurance funding) formula used in the Dutch national health insurance system adjusts only for age, gender, and location.[5] In the US, the HMO Medicare capitation formula adjusts for age, gender, welfare status, institutional status, and basis for Medicare eligibility (65+, disabled, end-stage renal disease). However, this formula contains no adjustments for functional health status or detailed levels of chronic illness.[6] Finally, Britain is about to introduce risk adjustment in its capitation formula for fundholding practices, but again the adjustments are likely to be only for age and gender.[7]

In light of the amount of risk adjustment in current capitation formulas, is risk selection likely to be profitable? To answer this question one must first recognize that, at most, 15 percent of the variance in individual-level data on year-to-year medical expenditures is predictable using observables. This empirical regularity has been verified by a number of researchers.[8] The potential for profits from risk selection exists, if the risk adjustment formula compensates for only a small fraction of these observables, while the insurer is successful in categorizing patients using a larger subset of these observables, and relies on them to risk select.

Van Vliet and van de Ven, using data from the Netherlands, have predicted the potential profits to be made from risk selection. Table 1 provides a summary of their statistical analysis using data on 20,000 individuals from the 1981 and 1982 Health Interview Surveys of the non-institutionalized population. The goal of the exercise was to see what factors (age, chronic conditions, etc.) could significantly predict a given patient's cost, and whether it was possible to predict more accurately than the risk-based funding provided by the government. To take a hypothetical example, the government's funding formula already provides larger payments for older individuals. If it is possible to predict that older asthmatics regularly cost more to insure then older non-asthmatics, and if the government funding does not already account for this, then risk selection can emerge. That is, insurers may try to enrol the non-asthmatic elderly and avoid asthma sufferers. The main statistical device for analyzing this possibility is the calculation of a "coefficient of variation," or R^2. The more variations in cost that a given set of characteristics can explain, the higher the R^2 will be. At the extreme, if R^2 was 100 percent, then whatever set of characteristics that were used to generate that R^2 could predict *exactly* how much a given patient would cost. In practice, however, previous researchers have demonstrated that a maximum of 15 percent of the variance in person-level data on year-to-year medical expenditures is predictable using readily available information on individual characteristics.[9]

In Model 1, Van Vliet and van de Ven include the list of risk adjusters currently used in the Dutch capitation formula, and obtain an R^2 of 2.8 percent. They add a supplemental set of sociodemographic characteristics in Model 2, which raises the R^2 to only 3.7 percent. However, reducing the number of sociodemographic indicators and adding instead an index of 25 chronic conditions (weighted by average medical consumption for each condition) dramatically raises the R^2 to 7.1 percent. Finally, including all the previous listed observables, plus a list of individuals' physical impairments and self-rated health, raises the R^2 to 11.4 percent — quite close to the maximum explainable variance of 15 percent.

Van Vliet and van de Ven assess the potential profits for risk selection by pointing out first that capitation payments in the Netherlands are calculated using a formula similar to Model 1. They consider the possibility that insurers collect all the data necessary to run a regression similar to Model 4 for their pool of applicants, and compute each individual's level of predicted expenditures. Each individual's predicted medical expenditures can then be compared to the capitation rate they would actually receive from the government (which uses Model 1), to determine whether the expected reimbursement rate is greater or less than expected costs. The authors find that good risks — those with predicted expenditures less than the capitation rate — have predicted costs on average 46 percent less than their capitation payment, while bad risks

Table 1
Explainable Variation
in Individual Medical Expenditures
Utilizing Dutch Data

Adjusters	Model 1	Model 2	Model 3	Model 4
Age/Sex Insurance Coverage Region	X	X	X	X
Employment Status Family Size		X	X	X
Socio-Economic Status Body Weight Degree of Urbanization Supply of Care Facilities Additional Insurance Coverage		X		X
Chronic Conditions (Weighted) Physical Impairments Self-rated General Health Status			X	X
Explained Variance (R^2 x 100)	2.8%	3.7%	7.1%	11.4%

SOURCE: R.C.J.A. Van Vliet and W.P.M.M. van de Ven, "Towards a Capitation Formula for Competing Health Insurers: An Empirical Analysis," *Social Science and Medicine*, Vol. 34, no. 9 (May 1992), pp. 1035-48.

have predicted costs on average 111 percent more than their capitation payment. Thus, insurers stand to gain a great deal from risk selection.

Similar results have been found using US data. Assuming mean annual Medicare expenditures of $3,000 per beneficiary, research finds that an HMO which can successfully explain one additional percentage point of medical expenditures over the capitation formula can gain $630 per enrollee.[10] If the HMO can successfully explain an additional 13 percentage points in medical expenditures, it will gain $1,530 per enrollee.

SOLUTIONS TO RISK SELECTION

Several solutions have been suggested to curb risk selection. Canada has avoided the problem by eliminating private insurers from the market and relying on the government as a universal insurer. In doing so, Canada experiences neither the advantages nor the disadvantages of internal markets.

In those countries that have already established internal markets or are considering adopting them, risk selection can be curbed through refinement of the capitation formulas. One of the potential instruments for refinement is an adjustment for individuals' prior use — for instance, medical expenditures in the previous year. The advantage of this adjuster is that it is easily measurable. However, prior use is also dependent upon existing provider practice styles, which may or may not be appropriate. Relying solely on prior use as an adjuster may inadvertently reward excessive treatment: if the payment for a patient goes up as a result of certain procedures being performed, that tends to encourage those procedures to be performed. Others recommend adjustment based on patients' existing chronic conditions. However, reporting these conditions may be subject to manipulation by insurers; for instance, insurers could have enrollees' blood pressure and pulse taken immediately after an exercise test in order to raise the apparent prevalence of hypertension in their casemix. Finally, van de Ven and Van Vliet suggest recursive refinement of capitation payments, in which regulators observe which patients are being denied access to insurance and augment their capitation ratios in subsequent periods.

Blended payment rates have been recommended by Newhouse as a means of moderating insurers' incentives to risk select.[11] These rates are a mixture of capitation and fee-for-service. Partial presence of capitation encourages providers to control health care costs, while fee-for-service reduces insurers' incentives to risk select. Finally, "risk corridors," in which profits or losses beyond a specified amount are shared by the insurer and the government, have also been suggested.[12] We still lack evidence on which of the above solutions is likely to work best in reducing risk selection. The plethora of potential solutions suggests that a workable one does indeed exist. Further experimentation with current and new systems of health care insurance is required to identify the optimal solution.

Finally, we must keep in mind that eliminating risk selection at the insurer level is no guarantee of optimal patient care. Capitation of providers can also lead *them* to engage in risk selection. For instance, health economists have demonstrated that capitated reimbursement according to Diagnosis Related Groups (DRGs) within the US Medicare programme gives hospitals an incentive to selectively treat relatively healthy patients within each DRG.[13]

Elimination of risk selection is not just a question of adjusting reimbursement rates. Pro-competitive regulation guaranteeing access and quality at the insurer *and* health care provider levels will also be required. If we are to pursue a system of internal markets, the remaining task will be to determine what mix of rate regulation and pro-competitive regulation is optimal for social welfare.

1. W. P. M. M. van de Ven and R. C. J. A. Van Vliet, "How Can We Prevent Cream Skimming in a Competitive Health Insurance Market? The Great Challenge for the 90's," in P. Zweifel and H. E. Frech III (eds.), *Developments in Health Economics and Public Policy: Health Economics Worldwide* (Boston: Kluwer Academic Publishers, 1992), pp. 23–46.

2. M. V. Pauly, "Is Cream-Skimming a Problem for the Competitive Medical Market?" *Journal of Health Economics,* Vol. 3 (1984), pp. 87–95.

3. P. Eggers, "Risk Differentials between Medicare Beneficiaries Enrolled and Not Enrolled in an HMO," *Health Care Financing Review,* (Winter 1980), pp. 91–99.

4. See van de Ven and Van Vliet, "How Can We Prevent Cream Skimming in a Competitive Health Insurance Market?"

5. R. C. J. A. Van Vliet and W. P. M. M. van de Ven, "Towards a Capitation Formula for Competing Health Insurers: An Empirical Analysis," *Social Science and Medicine,* Vol. 34, no. 9 (1992), pp. 1035–48.

6. J. P. Newhouse et al., "Adjusting Capitation Rates Using Objective Health Measures and Prior Utilization," *Health Care Financing Review,* Vol. 10, no. 3 (1989), pp. 41–54.

7. M. Matsaganis and H. Glennerster, "The Threat of Cream Skimming in the Post-Reform NHS," *Journal of Health Economics.* Vol. 13, no. 1 (March 1994), pp. 31–60.

8. W. P. Welch, "Regression toward the Mean in Medical Care Costs: Implications for Biased Selection in Health Maintenance Organizations," *Medical Care,* Vol. 23, no. 11 (1985), pp. 1234–41. See also Van Vliet and van de Ven, "Towards a Capitation Formula for Competing Health Insurers," and van de Ven and Van Vliet, "How Can We Prevent Cream Skimming in a Competitive Health Insurance Market?"

9. See Van Vliet and van de Ven, "Towards a Capitation Formula for

Competing Health Insurers"; Newhouse *et al.,* "Adjusting Capitation Rates Using Objective Health Measures and Prior Utilization"; and Welch, "Regression toward the Mean in Medical Care Costs."

10. See Newhouse *et al.,* "Adjusting Capitation Rates Using Objective Health Measures and Prior Utilization"; and also Van Vliet and van de Ven, "Towards a Capitation Formula for Competing Health Insurers."

11. J. P. Newhouse, "Pricing and Imperfections in the Medical Care Marketplace," in P. Zweifel and H. E. Frech III (eds.), *Developments in Health Economics and Public Policy: Health Economics Worldwide* (Boston: Kluwer Academic Publishers, 1992), pp. 3–22.

12. S. S. Wallack, C. P. Tompkins and L. Gruenberg, "A Plan for Rewarding Efficient HMOs," *Health Affairs,* Vol. 7 (1988), pp. 80–96.

13. D. Dranove, "Rate-Setting by Diagnosis Related Groups and Hospital Specialization," *Rand Journal of Economics,* Vol. 18, no. 3 (1987), pp. 417–27.

Å K E   B L O M Q V I S T

Reforming Health Care:

Canada and the Second Wave

Health Care Reform in International Perspective: The Second Wave

One of the most important developments in the industrialized world during the 20th century has been the emergence of "the welfare state": a range of social programmes to provide economic security for the citizenry. In all countries, reform of the systems for financing and producing health care services has played an important role in this process.

In continental Europe and Scandinavia, public sector programmes ensuring access to health services for broad segments of the population have a long history. In the English-speaking world, the most important early reform, at least from the viewpoint of distributional equity, was the establishment of the National Health Service (NHS) in Britain in the late 1940s. The most significant accomplishment of this reform was that it guaranteed every British citizen, without exception, access to the same comprehensive range of health services. Factors such as ability to pay or previous history of illness would no longer influence the comprehensiveness or cost of a person's insurance coverage or access to health services in times of illness.

Although the process would take another 25 years, by the early

1970s Canada had also achieved essentially universal coverage: by 1971, every province had a tax-financed programme[1] covering the cost of both hospital and physician services for its citizens, "on equal terms and conditions."

In the United States, universal coverage has not yet been achieved. However, Medicare and Medicaid programmes for those over 65 and those with low incomes were established in the 1960s. Thus, programmes to protect major segments of the population are an important feature of the US system as well, and the public sector share of total health care spending now exceeds 40 percent.

The process that began with the establishment of the NHS and ended in the early 1970s can be thought of as the "first wave" of health care reform. In the early 1990s, reform was once again high on the agenda in a number of countries.[2] Indeed, there are signs that the late 1980s represented the beginning of a second wave of reform. Not only the United States, but also the United Kingdom and a number of countries in continental Europe and Scandinavia, have been moving toward substantial restructuring of their systems of health care production and financing. Two recent publications that have the words "reform" and "health care" in their titles[3] include chapters on the following countries: Sweden, Holland, Germany, Belgium, France, Ireland, Spain, Canada, the UK and the US. To this list one could add Finland and possibly also Denmark, which has "hesitantly begun" a process of change (Saltman, in this volume).

In the first wave, the principal objective of reform was accessibility. In the second wave, in contrast, the emphasis is on the twin issues of cost control and efficiency. In most countries, aggregate health care expenditures, and public spending on health care, have grown considerably faster than other components of GDP during most of the post-war period. Although this does not necessarily mean that health care spending should be reined in,[4] in practice it has forced governments to implement increasingly effective measures to limit expenditure growth. As spending growth has slowed, the efficiency objective has become more prominent: when health care resources are more tightly controlled, it becomes more important to ensure that they are efficiently used. Moreover, efficiency does not relate only to the overall cost of production and administration in the health sector. In some countries, there has been dissatisfaction because of long waiting lists for certain kinds of medical care; the impersonal attitude and lack of concern, on the part of providers, for patient preferences (for example, to be treated by the same doctor or nurse on subsequent visits); and the perception of wide variation in treatment received, for similar conditions, at different clinics or hospitals. Calls for more efficiency in the health care sector may therefore relate to quality as well as cost.[5]

The Second Wave: What Are Its Elements?

In comparing the experience with formulating and implementing reform programmes in those countries where the second wave of reform is under way, or is at least being debated, one may distinguish several common elements in the strategies being pursued or proposed.

One common element is an emphasis on the advantages of increased *decentralization* of responsibility for resource allocation and management. I use the term in this context to refer to not only *geographical* but also *functional* decentralization (that is, giving more decision making power to administrative units responsible for specific functions).

Efforts at geographical decentralization have a long history in systems that originally were relatively centralized, such as those in the UK or the Canadian provinces. The presumption is that decentralization will lead not only to lower administration costs, but also to decision-making that is more sensitive to local needs and conditions and more responsive to patient preferences.

However, many in the health policy field have come to the view that such decentralization by itself is of limited effectiveness. In the recent debate, the emphasis has shifted to functional decentralization, in particular to the separation of responsibilities for *financing* and *purchasing* health services from that for *producing* them. Moreover, one may interpret past experience with decentralization as suggesting that the possibilities for enhancing efficiency by relying on administrative reforms within integrated bureaucracies are inherently limited.[6] For this reason, recent proposals have called for some form of "managed competition" among independently operating providers, or even different insurance plans.[7]

A second common theme in the new wave of reforms is the need to improve the appropriateness of care. Strategies include increased use of various forms of *managed care* and/or more emphasis on different kinds of formal *technology evaluation*.

A third element, finally, relates to the importance of patient freedom of choice among alternative providers and/or alternative insurance plans. This has played an especially important role in, on the one hand, Sweden, where the pre-reform system imposed severe restrictions on freedom of choice, and, on the other hand, the US, where many fear that universally available public insurance will mean reduced freedom of choice.[8]

Because the reform programmes discussed here envisage more reliance on competition and transactions based on contracts between buyers and sellers (of health services or health plans), they are often described as involving "markets." They have therefore revived an old question: what is the appropriate role of the market mechanism in the health care sector?

THE ROLE OF MARKETS IN THE HEALTH CARE SYSTEM: GENERAL CONSIDERATIONS

What role the market mechanism should play was, of course, a fundamental question during the debates preceding the first wave of health reform. At that time, the decision taken in most countries was to substantially *reduce* the role of the market mechanism in their existing financing and production systems. Their reasons generally had to do with the perception that, because of the special characteristics of health care as a commodity, the market mechanism would generally fail to do a good job of allocating resources in the health sector, even though it might perform acceptably in other sectors. A legitimate question concerning the recent proposals, therefore, is whether the arguments made against reliance on the market mechanism several decades ago do not continue to hold. That is, will an expanded role for some type of market mechanism not bring back precisely the kinds of inequity and inefficiency that the earlier reforms were supposed to eliminate?

Much of the opposition, at least in the popular debate, against the recent proposals is indeed based on this type of argument. Those like myself who advocate them, on the other hand, argue that the kinds of market-based arrangements now being proposed will be designed in such a way that the advantages gained in the first wave of reform will be preserved. In response to the objection that the problem of information asymmetry between buyer and seller necessarily renders the market mechanism ineffective in the health services industry,[9] the advocates of the proposals argue that modifications in the system of remunerating health services producers can be used to overcome this problem.

More importantly, the fundamental deficiency of a market for private insurance, from the viewpoint of both efficiency and distributional equity, is the complex and discriminatory structure of premium setting and risk classification that it tends to produce. None of the recent proposals would involve such a system: to be taken seriously, any reform proposal in Europe or Canada must preserve the basic principle that everyone, regardless of factors such as income or risk of illness, should have access to adequate health services in times of need.[10] That is, the equity-based commitment to universal access must remain. Although the term "internal markets" is used by different people to mean somewhat different things, an important function of the modifier "internal" is to suggest that the proposals involve the use of market-based arrangements *within a system in which the basic parameters have been set by government,* and in which it can be taken as understood that the equity principle will not be compromised.

I will now turn to the question of how and to what extent reforms of the internal market type could be used to improve the Canadian health care system.

INTERNAL MARKETS: A CANADIAN PERSPECTIVE

As Maynard (this volume) puts it, a market is a network of buyers and sellers. Using this definition in a broad sense, one may argue that the present Canadian health care system already involves "markets" to a substantial extent. Physician services (both primary and specialist care) are "bought" directly by patients from individual doctors, even though in each province they are entirely paid for by a single insurance plan, on the basis of a uniform fee-for-service schedule negotiated, by the government, with the provincial medical associations.[11] Similarly, Canadian acute care hospitals are technically private, non-profit institutions, with their own boards of directors. The hospital system in each province may therefore be considered a "network of sellers" from which the provincial government buys hospital services on behalf of the citizens; in this case, the transaction involves a global budget negotiated separately between the government and each hospital.

Thus, even though many people, especially in the US, consider the

Canadian health care system to be part of the public sector, one may also argue, as Raisa Deber does,[12] that it is more properly characterized as a system with public funding but private provision. This contrasts with the pre-reform system in the UK, under which hospital and specialist physician services were provided directly by the NHS in hospitals that it owned and by doctors who were NHS employees; similarly, under the pre-reform Swedish system, hospitals were owned and operated directly by the county councils *(landsting),* who were responsible for financing the health care system and who were the employers of most physicians, both hospital-based specialists and those providing primary care.

Deber's characterization and the description of the Canadian system of funding hospitals as a "market" are both somewhat arbitrary, of course. One might argue, for example, that a non-profit institution that can sell its services only to a single public sector buyer is not really a "private" institution. By the same token, a hospital that derives its revenue on the basis of an annual global budget negotiated with the government is not "selling its services in a market" any more than a government department that depends for its funding on an annually negotiated budget is participating in a market. Both the "public *versus* private" and the "market *versus* non-market" distinctions are, in reality, multidimensional ones: factors such as the extent of competition among service providers, or the incentive structure inherent in the system of paying for the services provided, may be at least as important in predicting the efficiency with which the system will operate. Thus, even though the present Canadian health care system already has some of the characteristics being introduced or proposed in the European systems (in particular, a high degree of decentralization of health services production), it lacks other features that are fundamental to the European reforms (e.g., with respect to competition and incentive structures).

Will market-based health care reform be a serious item on the Canadian political agenda in the medium term? The answer is not clear. On the one hand, there is an entrenched view in Canada that we should not tinker with our health care system: it already does an admirable job, providing universal access to quality care at a much lower cost than the US, where universal access has *not* been achieved. Those who hold this view tend to interpret concepts like "internal markets" and "competition" as suggesting that the types of reform being advocated would make our system similar to the American.

On the other hand, international statistics indicate that Canada has recently become only the second country ever to devote as much as 10 percent of its GDP to health care[13] — this even though the age structure of Canada's population is relatively favourable. (In a number of comparable European countries the elderly population is proportionately much larger.) In the words of Bill Tholl,[14] although Canada does not have the most expensive system, it has become the international "silver medallist health spender," with an apparent cost-effectiveness performance poorer than that of the major publicly funded systems in Europe. On top of this, Canada is fast approaching a public-finance crisis: its debt-deficit position, especially when the federal and provincial governments are taken together, is worse than that of most OECD countries. In the circumstances, one cannot expect health, which, next to education, is the largest single expenditure category in the public sector, to escape the pressure for cost reductions and efficiency improvements.

Although a variety of policy initiatives have been under way for some time in the provinces,[15] these have not involved any fundamental changes to the system of funding and service production; it can be argued that they have been aimed more at cost containment than at efficiency improvement. In the following pages I will consider a recently published, relatively radical set of proposals that involves an application of some of the principles in the European reform movement that could be adapted for Canada. Henceforth, I will refer to them as the Blomqvist/Brown/Soderstrom proposals.[16]

THEME I: DECENTRALIZATION OF FUNDING

Since any market involves sales and purchases, proposals for reforms based on internal markets can be analyzed by answering a modified version of the tripartite question familiar to anyone who has studied elementary microeconomics: *Who* is supposed to buy *What,* and *from Whom?*[17]

In the case of functional decentralization, whereby some kind of "funding agency" would buy health services on behalf of its clients in an internal market, the answer is very general: *Who* is the public funding agency, *What* is the full range of health services, and *Whom* is the independent producers of health services. As noted, the Canadian system already incorporates a version of this principle: responsibility for funding rests with the provincial government, while responsibility for services production has been delegated to a substantial extent to individual physicians and hospitals. However, in each province there is a high degree of geographical centralization of the funding/purchasing function, and — at least in the larger provinces — it appears likely that substantial efficiency gains could be made by geographically decentralizing the funding function currently carried out by the provincial ministries of health.

In centralized systems, certain regions of a province may, for historical or political reasons, end up with a share of the health care budget out of proportion to their population or, more generally, to some index of the "need" for services. For example, in Canada it is often argued that the larger cities receive more than their share, even when account is taken of their specialized facilities that are supposed to serve outlying areas as well. In a decentralized system, financing authorities in outlying areas would agree to "buy" services from urban facilities only if this were cheaper than providing them locally, and only in the quantities really required locally.[18] Another argument in favour of decentralization is the general presumption that local decision makers are in a more appropriate position to adapt to local conditions and preferences.

Proposals for this type of decentralization are not new: systems of "population-based funding" have been advocated by Evans,[19] among others, and are being actively studied by the government of Ontario. Under such a system, funds for health services production would be allocated to local units, similar to the British District Health Authorities, on the basis of some type of adjusted population count.[20] These units would be free to spend their budgets as they saw fit, but would have formal responsibility for purchasing (contracting for) health services of acceptable quality for the population in their jurisdiction. *What* in this case could be either hospital services only, or both hospital and physician services. The objective of producing good health using the most efficient mix of physician services and hospital services strongly suggests that the same local agency should ultimately have responsibility for the cost of both services.

As Swedish and British experience indicates, an important aspect of the *What* question concerns the specification of the seller's responsibility under the contract, and the basis of payment. It would be possible to decentralize without changing the present system of funding hospitals on the basis of individually negotiated global budgets; however, this system has the weakness that it does not specify in detail what the hospital's responsibilities are, beyond an implicit commitment to provide quality care to as many patients as possible. Efficiency gains might be made by negotiating more explicit contracts: precisely what range of services each hospital must provide, for what client population and in what numbers. Indeed, such contracts would be necessary to the extent that some funding agencies would negotiate for certain specialized services in facilities located outside their jurisdictions (see below).

Moreover, with more explicit contracts there may well be additional efficiency gains to be had from modifying the basis on which hospitals are paid. For example, they might be paid through some form of Diagnosis Related Groupings (DRGs), or through some form of "block contract" or capitation. Many alternatives are possible; I will return to the issue in more detail below in the context of the extent to which it might be desirable to base the system on the principle of "managed care." In some cases it may also be appropriate to let hospitals charge on a fee-for-service basis, with itemized bills (e.g., for rarely performed services or for patients from other jurisdictions).

With respect to the question *from Whom?*, a critical issue is the extent to which the funding agency should be allowed to purchase services from producers (such as hospitals) in other jurisdictions. A fundamental idea behind the concept of internal markets is that it can be used to introduce competition — or at least potential competition — among sellers, and that this can act as an incentive to contain costs or, more generally, to promote efficiency. Potential competition is, of course, enhanced if each funding agency is allowed to purchase a wide range of services from sellers both outside and within their jurisdiction.

It should be noted, finally, that geographical decentralization along the lines recommended in the Blomqvist/Brown/Soderstrom proposals implies some restrictions on the patient's freedom to choose provider — whereas under the present system one is free to seek care from any physician and, effectively, from any hospital in one's province of residence.[21] Under a system that bases provision on negotiated contracts between providers and local funding agencies, some limits would have to be placed on patients' right to seek care from providers not covered by a contract with "their" agency. A partial solution can be found in the system used by some US Preferred Provider Organizations (PPOs) or Health Maintenance Organizations (HMOs), under which patients who seek care from "outside" providers must pay for the cost of this care, over and above some preset amount. However, this solution presupposes a modification of the current Canadian policy under which providers are not allowed to collect any fee from patients. I will return to this issue in discussing the principle of managed care as part of a Canadian reform programme.

Some Practical Considerations

In the debate over decentralization and contract-based care, there are sceptics who, while not questioning the logic of the principles involved, argue that in practice the effectiveness of such a system will be limited by a number of factors not considered in the theoretical analysis.

One objection is that, in places with little excess capacity, funding agencies would have no choice but to sign contracts with all existing facilities. Conversely, it is argued that in the opposite situation, in which there *is* excess capacity, funding agencies would find it politically impossible to actually close down a hospital that could not offer an attractive contract. Why, the critics ask, would one expect local funding agencies to be any more capable of bringing about a more efficient allocation of hospital resources, say, than provincial officials under the present system?

These criticisms certainly have merit, and they draw attention to a number of practical issues such as how the officials in the local funding agencies would be chosen. (In Blomqvist/Brown/Soderstrom it is argued that, in order to emphasize their public accountability, these officials should be chosen in local elections.) These criticisms are also consistent with Swedish experience so far, which indicates that in the short run there is considerable inertia in the system: functional decentralization has not made a great deal of difference in terms of how money has been allocated, since buying agencies have mostly signed "non-specific block contracts" with existing suppliers (the phrase is from Saltman in this volume).

Nevertheless, in the long run the combination of geographical and functional decentralization could have a substantial impact. As previously noted, geographical decentralization in the form of population-based funding would provide an automatic and powerful incentive to investigate whether efficiency could be improved by reducing regional and local imbalances in distribution of facilities. In addition, an important potential benefit of contract negotiations would be the generation of a better information base on the cost of different kinds of care and services in different facilities. On the one hand, institutional managers would have greater incentive to generate accurate cost information in order to bid on contracts. On the other hand, individual funding agencies would be able to use information from contracts in other areas to gauge the reasonableness of the bids they receive. Better cost information might not lead to drastic action (such as hospital closings) in the short run; it could, however, serve as the basis for the decisions regarding investment and re-investment of capital resources that, in the long run, determine the distribution of institutional services.

I will now turn to the second major theme in health care reform in a number of countries: the introduction of some form of managed care.

THEME II: MANAGED CARE

The concept of managed care refers to the idea that, in seeking treatment during the course of an illness, a patient will be able to use particular services only with the prior approval of whoever acts as "manager." In the US, the concept often describes insurance arrangements that require second opinions or prior approval before certain services will be covered (or arrangements whereby the insurer directly decides what services will be provided, as in the case of insurance through an HMO); it has also been used in the Medicaid plans of certain states. In other countries, particularly the UK, managed care may take the form of assigning a "gatekeeping" function to a primary care physician whose referral is required before institutional or specialist care can be provided.

Evidence from the US suggests that managed care can produce substantial cost savings when compared to an open-ended, conventional, fee-for-service system. At the same time, British experience is consistent with the idea that managed care can be a useful adjunct to global cost controls in the design of a publicly financed system that provides good health care at reasonable cost.

Managed Care and Internal Markets

Managed care may, of course, be used even in a system that is not organized around internal markets. For example, in the pre-reform British system, GPs were expected to perform a gatekeeping function with respect to hospital and specialist services, even though these services were not provided in internal markets.[22] Nevertheless, internal markets and managed care can be seen as complementary elements in promoting efficiency.

On the one hand, care management is likely to be more effective in a market system. As noted, one of the consequences of greater reliance on internal markets is awareness of and information about the cost of producing various health services — since these costs will be the basis for negotiations on service contracts between producers and funding agencies. With better information on the cost of different services, it will be easier to assess the impact of care management on the cost of dealing with particular illnesses, or providing health care to particular population groups.

On the other hand, managed care could greatly enhance the ability of an internal market system to improve efficiency in the system as a whole. While contract negotiations between providers and funding agencies may help reduce the unit cost of producing particular services, it provides neither the incentive nor the responsibility to use the most cost-effective *combination* of services in dealing with particular health problems. For example, substitution may be possible between physician and hospital services, between diagnostic and curative services, between surgical and medical treatment, and so on, when dealing with a given illness. Given such substitution possibilities, efficiency might be greatly enhanced by the services of a well-informed decision maker, who would be responsible for choosing the most cost-effective course of action and who would have an incentive for doing so.

The issues involved here can be related to one of the oldest and most hotly debated questions in health economics — "how to pay the doctor." The high cost of conventional fee-for-service systems is often explained by the fact that under them physicians have no monetary incentive to make decisions that save money for the system as a whole. Their only incentive is to ensure that their patients receive "the best available care, regardless of cost," and the more of their own services they provide, the higher their income. Patients, even if they were to have an incentive to save (which they do not, under the Canadian system of zero user charges), would in any case not be sufficiently informed to make the necessary decisions.

The incentive for cost-increasing "supplier-induced demand" under a conventional fee-for-service system can be counteracted in one or both of the following ways: by changing the incentive structure for physicians, who effectively make the treatment decisions; or by creating mechanisms by which to monitor the number of services used in each treatment episode (that is, some form of managed care). HMOs sometimes employ both: the physicians are often salaried, and their treatment decisions are subject to internal rules and guidelines designed to promote cost effectiveness.[23] Various ways of monitoring physicians and hospitals are also used in American private sector managed-care arrangements, such as PPOs. British GPs have no incentive to "over-provide" services since they are paid by a combination of salary and capitation (that is, an amount that depends on the number of patients signed up on their list during a given month); similarly, specialists are paid by salary. In addition, GPs act as care managers in that their referral is required in order for a patient to have access to hospital and specialist care. Moreover, the 1989 British reforms introduced the GP "fundholding option," which was designed as an *incentive* for GPs to fulfil their care management responsibility.

Introducing Managed Care in Canada

How could managed care be introduced into a reformed Canadian system? In Blomqvist/Brown/Soderstrom it is argued that the simplest way would be through a version of the British GP system, under which each citizen would have to be registered with a primary care physician, such as a family doctor, whose referral would be required for access to other health services and who would have formal responsibility for the care of patients on her or his list.

The logic of care management dictates that the managing agent should not be paid on a fee-for-service basis, but instead through salary or capitation. Recent Swedish experience illustrates that the salary alternative raises the question of what to do with those doctors who do not attract a large number of patients. Conversely, a system of reimbursement based at least in part on capitation has the advantage of creating a link between the revenue and the productivity of an individual care manager (the more patients a doctor assumes responsibility for, the higher her or his income). Moreover, provided patients have the right to choose their care manager, it also rewards productivity in that it gives doctors an incentive to respond to patients' treatment preferences.

There is also a strong theoretical argument for "putting care managers at risk" — that is, making them responsible for some of the cost of drugs, hospital services, etc., that their patients receive on their referral. The UK fundholding reform is a step in that direction, even though its effectiveness may be limited by the fact that care managers do not directly benefit from any surplus they manage to create; nor is it clear precisely what happens to GPs who exceed their budget.[24] In any case, valuable evidence on how an effective system of fundholding can be designed will become available as data from the British experiments accumulate, and could be used in designing a Canadian version.

Introduction of a system of managed care along these lines would to some extent modify the role envisaged for the local funding agencies in negotiating service contracts with providers. Specifically, it affects in two ways the *What* part of the *Who, What,* and *from Whom?* question. On the one hand, funding agencies would be buying not only primary care services but also "care management" — from family doctors and others. On the other hand, it is not *a priori* obvious how responsibility should be divided between care managers and local funding agencies in negotiating with providers of other types of care, such as hospitals. Since care managers would act as referring agents, a strong case can be made for allowing them to establish referral networks on terms negotiated with the hospitals; the argument is especially strong if the care managers would pay part of the cost of their patients' institutional care. Clearly, however, these contracts would have to be taken into account in the negotiations between hospitals and the funding agencies who pay most of their cost. Solutions to these contracting problems should not be beyond human ingenuity; at the same time, however, the transactions costs associated with finding them should not be under-estimated.

Another form of managed care that has been discussed in some Canadian provinces and that might involve lower transactions costs of this type is referred to as the Comprehensive Health Organization (CHO). Modelled on the American HMOs, CHOs would, in return for capitation payments, be responsible for providing both primary and other forms of care to their populations.[25] Both forms could exist together, and consumers in communities served by both could have the right to enrol either in a CHO or with a family doctor. Needless to say, the expectation would be that competition between the two forms would tend to promote efficiency.[26]

A system with an option to choose either CHOs or primary care providers such as family doctors would represent a hybrid of, on the one hand, the UK reform package and, on the other, the reforms proposed in Holland. Under the Dekker proposals, all Dutch citizens would have to sign up with a "care insurer" responsible for providing a comprehensive package of health services to its clients; the role of the (single) funding agency would be limited to negotiating the terms of the contracts offered by the care insurer to its enrollees.[27] The role envisaged for a CHO would be similar to that of a care insurer: the *What* that either one would be selling to a funding agency would be a comprehensive insurance package.

A Digression on Technology Evaluation and Quality Monitoring

One of the best-established findings in recent health policy research is that many technologies have come into widespread use even though there has been little or no systematic evaluation of their medical effectiveness, let alone their cost effectiveness. In some cases, ineffective technologies have continued to be used long after their ineffectiveness has been established.[28] A related, equally well-established finding is that in a number of countries there is at any given time a great deal of variation in how different medical practitioners treat similar categories of patients and health problems.[29] Both of these findings suggest that there are substantial efficiency gains to be had from (1) more systematic evaluation of the medical and cost effectiveness of existing and new technologies, and (2) measures to reduce the variability in practice patterns among doctors so as to bring them closer to the most cost-effective pattern.

The issue of appropriate use of technology is usually considered independently of health care reform. However, I will argue that the introduction of incentive-based internal markets may serve to reduce the scope of problems in this regard. Another consequence may be a greater need for more systematic techniques for defining and monitoring the quality of care.

Incentives and Technology

Even though problems with respect to practice variations and technology evaluation have been apparent for some time, it is fair to say that in the US and Canada progress in overcoming them has been slow. Attempts at providing better information to doctors do not seem to have been very effective in reducing practice variability,[30] and new technologies are still being adopted before their effectiveness has been established. On the other hand, there is evidence to suggest that in the UK part of the reason for the relatively low per capita cost of care can be attributed to the existence and enforcement of stricter rules governing the use of expensive medical technologies than those in North America.[31]

To what should this difference be ascribed? One plausible suggestion has to do with incentive structures. In the fee-for-service North American systems, doctors (and hospitals) have little economic incentive to strive for cost effectiveness. The only agent with such an interest is the third-party payer, but, until the recent advent of managed care, private insurance companies were reluctant to challenge the principle of "clinical autonomy" — that is, that the physician should not be subject to restrictions of any kind when deciding how a patient is to be treated. The weak incentives to seek the most cost-effective care may have translated into a lack of demand for systematic technology evaluation and for research into ways of finding cheaper, more cost-effective technologies.[32]

In a system under which managed care plays a major role, and under which the care manager is paid through some form of capitation or (in the case of gatekeeping primary care-givers) capitation *cum* fundholding, there *is* an incentive to stay abreast of research. It is in a manager's interest to know which technologies are ineffective and should be abandoned, and to exploit quickly new technologies that can treat particular conditions at lower cost than existing methods.

The demand for cost-effective technology may also serve to attract the resources (both private and public) to research aimed at *developing* such technology. In the long run, this effect may be even more crucial to promoting efficiency than the fact that capitation involves an incentive to *use* the least expensive technology among those whose relative cost effectiveness is already known.

Incentives and the Quality of Care

By the same token, however, it should be recognized that the incentive structure under capitation, or capitation *cum* fundholding, may produce a different kind of inefficiency: it may serve as an incentive to save by providing low-quality care, especially if it is difficult for the patient to monitor quality; or to under-provide care, especially if it is difficult for the patient or an outside agent to ascertain whether additional care would have been beneficial.[33] For this reason, a system dominated by capitation as the mode of payment may require measures to strengthen the ability of the patient's agent — that is, the funding agency — to systematically monitor quality. (This is just the mirror image of the monitoring for *over-provision* that might be required in a system dominated by fee-for-service.) In addition, new legal approaches may need to be developed to facilitate specification and enforcement of quality control of contracted care.[34]

Theme III: Internal Markets and Freedom of Choice

The third feature common to current reform proposals is an emphasis on preserving or strengthening patient freedom of choice. From a Canadian viewpoint, this is an especially important issue: one of the perceived strengths of the Canadian system is that it has succeeded in ensuring equal access to care *without* paying the price, in terms of restricting the freedom to choose provider, that has been paid to some extent in the UK and particularly in the pre-reform Swedish system. It is even more important in light of the ideological significance of the freedom-of-choice issue in the American debate: to a Canadian, the oft-repeated claim in the US that a system of "socialized medicine" such as Canada's necessarily implies less freedom of choice appears misleading at best.

There is no denying that in some ways the kind of reform advocated above can be interpreted as reducing freedom of choice. By definition, a system of managed care restricts patients to the services dispensed by those providers to whom they have been referred by their care manager. By the same token, a system of contracts negotiated between providers and local funding agencies can be effective only if it implies some restrictions on patients' rights to obtain services from providers with whom their agencies do not have contracts.[35]

The freedom to choose among providers is, however, only one dimension of the attractiveness of a public health insurance system. Another is cost. If a reform package of the type outlined in Blomqvist/Brown/Soderstrom were to significantly reduce the average cost of care to the taxpayer, most people might consider the reduced freedom of choice as a price worth paying. Moreover, patients would have the right to choose their managing agent (primary care-giver or, possibly, CHO), as they do under the UK system.[36] Another possibility would be to allow patients to obtain care, on payment of a surcharge, from providers other than those approved by their care managers.

Many observers would argue that a drawback of the Canadian system is that while it offers unrestricted choice of provider, it offers no choice with respect to alternative forms of insurance. For example, many people might prefer to be insured through a system with a deductible, or under a system of managed care, if they had that option and if the lower expected costs under such policies were to be reflected in premium reductions.[37] In Canada, any such alternative insurance options would be controversial since they might be seen as conflicting with the equity objective — the argument being that they would be most attractive to consumers at low risk of illness, whose relative welfare would increase in comparison to those at high risk. However, provided the standard of care of those staying with the full-coverage option remained unchanged (through increased government subsidies, if necessary), I do not share this objection: my personal view is that the equity objective essentially represents a commitment to protect the *absolute* standards of those with a low real income.

CONCLUSION

The idea of using internal market mechanisms as an element in Canadian health care reform is bound to be controversial. To repeat: a fundamental feature of the Canadian health policy debate is the conviction that because our system is better than the American one we should not do anything that would make our system resemble theirs. In the popular debate, the idea of "markets" tends to be identified with the US system, and thus something that we should stay away from.

Canadian reaction to the increasing use of market-based concepts in European health care reform is somewhat mixed. On the one hand, there are those who see it as a sign of a weakening European commitment to equity in health policy (and in social policy in general), a trend they believe Canada should resist. On the other hand, there are those who interpret the European willingness to use the market mechanism as evidence of a welcome distinction between ends and means in health policy: as long as the *objectives* are set in a way that preserves the commitment to equity, the mechanisms used to accomplish them can be pragmatically designed and be based on efficiency criteria. Needless to say, my own sympathies go in the latter direction. Indeed, I take the view that given Canada's present public finance predicament, a commitment to equity will in the end *force* us to improve the efficiency of our health care and our other social programmes.

It must also be admitted, however, that anyone who argues in favour of reforms based on internal markets at the present time does so largely on faith. The amount of hard evidence on whether, in reality, internal market reforms would lead to substantial efficiency gains (net of transactions costs) is still very limited. Indeed, given the argument that a large portion of the potential gains are likely to be long-term, this is not surprising: there is no country in which internal markets have been operating effectively for a long time. More empirical research would obviously be welcome, and will no doubt be forthcoming.

Finally, it must be noted that the above discussion has not touched on one aspect that inevitably will play a major part in the debate on health care reform in Canada — namely, the division of responsibility for health policy between the federal and provincial levels of government.[38] In my view, the dynamics of the Canadian political process in recent years have been a detriment to health policy reform: attempts by the provincial governments who manage the system to experiment with policy innovations have been hampered by dogmatic and simplistic attitudes toward health policy among federal politicians.[39] However, fiscal pressures and other forces impinging on the political process in Canada may gradually change this, and move serious health care reform to a higher position on the policy agenda.

1. While some provinces imposed what was referred to as "health insurance premiums" to finance part of the cost of the programmes, to the extent that these premiums were uniform and compulsory they were in effect just another form of taxation.

2. Although the focus here is on industrialized countries, health reform in the developing world was also becoming an important topic in the 1980s and 1990s. For an extended discussion, see World Bank, *World Development Report 1993: Investing in Health* (Washington, DC: World Bank, 1993).

3. See Chris Ham, Ray Robinson and Michaela Benzeval, *Health Check: Health Care Reforms in an International Context* (London: King's Fund Institute, 1990); and Organisation for Economic Co-operation and Development, *The Reform of Health Care: A Comparative Analysis of Seven OECD Countries,* Health Policy Studies, No. 2 (Paris: OECD, 1992).

4. Technically, it is possible that the income elasticity of health care demand is greater than one, in which case it is optimal for the sector's share of aggregate resources to rise with rising incomes. Or, as more sophisticated technological opportunities arise over time, it may be efficient (contribute more to human welfare) to increase the share of total resources spent on health.

5. In the US, the distinction between the two phases of health reform does not fit as well as in other countries, of course, because universality of coverage has not yet been achieved. Nevertheless, since the aggregate cost of health care relative to GDP is considerably higher in the US than in any other country, there is as much interest in the issue of cost control there as elsewhere, and the argument has been made that the objectives of universality of coverage and of efficiency improvements in the US system are inextricably linked: the chances of achieving universal coverage might be considerably improved if Congress and the public can be convinced that it can be financed in part through savings resulting from more efficient methods of production

and administration in the health sector.

6.   Although the structure of the British NHS provided for a considerable degree of decentralization by the mid-1980s, it could still be considered an integrated bureaucracy, and the view that substantial inefficiencies remained in the way in which it was administered ultimately led to the shift toward functional decentralization characteristic of the reform proposals of 1989. Similarly, efforts to improve efficiency through decentralizing some of the decision-making powers of provincial governments to local advisory bodies in the Canadian provinces have met with at most limited success. For a discussion of the Canadian case, see Canadian Medical Association, *The Language of Health System Reform: Report of the Working Group on Regionalization and Decentralization* (Ottawa: CMA, 1993).

7.   I am using the term "insurance plan" in this context to refer to the "care insurers" or "health plans" that form the basis for the Dutch reform proposals in the Dekker Plan or the original Clinton Plan for US reform.

8.   Paradoxically, the issue of freedom for the patient to choose provider has become more important to many Americans because of the increasing prevalence of managed care plans in the *private* sector; as further discussed below, such plans necessarily imply at least some restrictions on this freedom.

9.   The information asymmetry problem is perhaps the main factor emphasized by those health economists who argue that competitive markets have failed in the past. For a forceful statement of this position, see Robert G. Evans, *Strained Mercy: The Economics of Canadian Health Care* (Toronto: Butterworths, 1984).

10.   Once again, the case of the US is a bit different, of course. Although the original Clinton Plan is based on a form of internal markets for health insurance *and* universal access, it now appears likely that whatever reform package is ultimately adopted (if any) it will not achieve universality. However, unless its original intent is completely subverted as it winds its tortuous way through Congress, it should come closer to universality than the present system.

11.   Alternatively, one might consider the insurance plan itself as the "buyer" of physician services, on behalf of the insured patients. In

Canada, where federal legislation essentially prohibits any out-of-pocket charges to patients, this viewpoint might even seem the more natural one. On the other hand, Canadian patients are, of course, "buyers" in the sense that the transactions take place at their initiative, with no requirement for prior approval from the provincial plan; see below.

12. See Raisa B. Deber, G. Ross Baker and Sharmila L. Mhatre, "Review of Provincial Systems," in S. Mathwin Davies (ed.), *Health Care: Innovation, Impact, and Challenge* (Kingston, Ont.: Queen's University School of Public Administration and School of Policy Studies, 1992).

13. See William G. Tholl, "Health Care Spending in Canada: Skating Faster on Thinner Ice," in Åke G. Blomqvist and David M. Brown (eds.), *Limits to Care: Reforming Canada's Health System in an Age of Restraint* (Toronto: C. D. Howe Institute, 1994), pp. 53–89.

14. See Tholl, "Health Care Spending in Canada," p. 78.

15. See Raisa B. Deber, G. Ross Baker and Sharmila L. Mhatre, "A Review of Provincial Initiatives," in Åke G. Blomqvist and David M. Brown (eds.), *Limits to Care: Reforming Canada's Health System in an Age of Restraint* (Toronto: C. D. Howe Institute, 1994), pp. 91–124; and Ontario Hospital Association, *Restructuring Canada's Health Care System: Provincial Overviews* (Toronto: Ontario Hospital Association, 1993).

16. See Blomqvist and Brown (eds.), *Limits to Care.* In addition to the chapters by Blomqvist, pp. 3–50 and pp. 399-432, in which a specific set of proposals is summarized, alternative types of market-based reforms are extensively discussed in the chapter by Lee Soderstrom, pp. 217–65. The chapter by Bradford L. Kirkman-Liff, pp. 167–216, contains a systematic survey of the reform proposals in Holland, Germany and the UK on which the Blomqvist/Brown/Soderstrom proposals draw. A brief summary is also provided in Åke G. Blomqvist, *Sound Advice: Prescriptions for Health Care Reform in Canada,* C. D. Howe Institute Commentary, no. 58 (Toronto: C. D. Howe Institute, 1994).

17. For those who have not looked at an elementary micro text recently, the original tripartite question, referring to the way in which a society should use its scarce resources, is: *What* (should be produced)? *How*

(that is, using what resource combinations, should different commodities be produced)? *For Whom* (should the goods be produced; that is, how should income be distributed)?

18. Note that in a decentralized system of this kind there would necessarily have to be at least some degree of functional decentralization as well, to the extent that local agencies decide to buy certain services from jurisdictions other than their own. Note also that decentralized funding would of necessity have to be accompanied by some restrictions on patients' right to seek treatment outside their own jurisdiction. These issues are further discussed below.

19. See Robert G. Evans, "Health Care Reform: The Issue from Hell," *Policy Options,* Vol. 14, no. 6 (July-August 1993), pp. 35–41.

20. The adjustments to the population base would, at a minimum, reflect differences in age composition, since age is an important determinant of health needs. The extent to which other factors influencing "need" should be incorporated is a controversial issue. In particular, there is controversy over whether and to what extent historical cost differences should be taken into account.

21. Indeed, since each province's insurance plan is "portable" (that is, provides for coverage when a person is in another province), a person can, in principle, seek care from any provider in Canada.

22. The term "managed care" is an American one of relatively recent origin, and since the normal usage of the term in the contemporary US debate refers to situations in which the care manager has a financial incentive to keep the costs of treatment down, it may be objected that it cannot be applied to the pre-reform British system: under that system, GPs had no direct financial incentive to be efficient in performing the gatekeeping function, since they were not responsible for any part of the cost of the services their patients received following their referrals. Moreover, GPs could not ensure that their patients would in fact receive the hospital and specialist services that they recommended, since such services were rationed.

    In my view, it may nevertheless be argued that the referral decisions of British GPs in the pre-reform system were similar to those that a contemporary American care manager has to make: in both cases, the objective is to decide whether a particular patient's need for a particular procedure is great enough to justify the cost (in the US case, the direct cost to the third-party payer; in the British case, the cost in the form of using up valuable hospital services or specialist consultation).

23.   A general term used in the US to denote incentive structures that overcome the incentive toward "supplier-induced demand" is Prospective Payments Systems, PPS. The DRG system used in US Medicare is another example.

24.   In assessing the degree of risk to which fundholding GPs are subject, it is important to note that the costs for which they are potentially responsible refer only to a specified set of "elective" hospital procedures. This of course gives them more ability to control hospital costs than they would have if the budgets had referred to non-elective procedures as well.

25.   An ambitious effort to create a CHO based on a large Toronto hospital at present appears to be stalled due to administrative problems. However, plans to create experimental CHOs in several smaller Ontario communities are under way.

26.   Managed care also is a key element in the reform proposals developed independently by Monique Jérôme-Forget and Claude E. Forget, "Internal Markets in the Canadian Context," pp. 193-218 in this volume. From a technical point of view, their TMAs (Targeted Medical Agencies) are similar to fundholding primary care managers, although it is envisaged that they will consist of physicians practising as a group.

Jérôme-Forget and Forget do not favour management through organizations such as CHOs or HMOs, on the grounds that such large organizations will inevitably develop into cumbersome and costly bureaucracies. While I sympathize with this concern, I believe that such bureaucracies are to some extent inevitable in a system where some way has to be found to manage large hospitals, and the marginal administrative cost of adding care management responsibilities to such organizations may not be very high. Moreover, if CHOs have to compete for clients with primary care fundholders, they will not survive unless they are as successful in meeting patient preferences as the latter.

27.   Note that the role of the "care insurers" in the Dekker Plan bears a

strong resemblance to that envisaged for the "health plans" in which Americans would be enrolled under the original Clinton Plan.

28. See David Feeny, "Technology Assessment and Health Policy in Canada," in Blomqvist and Brown (eds.), *Limits to Care,* pp. 295–326.

29. For a review of the small-area variations (SAV) literature, see Peter C. Coyte, "Providers' Perceptions, Geographic Variations, and the Cost-Effective Provision of Health Care Services," in Blomqvist and Brown (eds.), *Limits to Care,* pp. 269–94.

30. Jonathan Lomas *et al.,* "Do Practice Guidelines Guide Practice? The Effect of a Consensus Statement on the Practice of Physicians," *New England Journal of Medicine,* Vol. 321 (1989), pp. 1306–11.

31. A fascinating discussion of this issue can be found in H. J. Aaron and W. B. Schwartz, *The Painful Prescription: Rationing Hospital Care* (Washington, DC: The Brookings Institution, 1984).

32. For theoretical analyses that stress these factors, see John H. Goddeeris, "Insurance and Incentives for Innovation in Medical Care," *Southern Economic Journal,* Vol. 51 (1984), pp. 530–39; and "Medical Insurance, Technological Change, and Welfare," *Economic Inquiry,* Vol. 22 (1984), pp. 56–57. See also James R. Baumgardner, "The Interaction between Forms of Insurance Contracts and Types of Technological Change in Health Care," *Rand Journal,* Vol. 22 (1991), pp. 36–53. For a survey, see also Burton A. Weisbrod, "The Health Care Quadrilemma: An Essay on Technological Change, Insurance, Quality of Care, and Cost Containment," *Journal of Economic Literature,* Vol. 29 (1991), pp. 523–52.

33. For a formal analysis, see Åke G. Blomqvist, "The Doctor as Double Agent: Information Asymmetry, Health Insurance, and Medical Care," *Journal of Health Economics,* Vol. 10 (1991), pp. 411–32.

34. The logic discussed here raises the question: would one not expect American HMOs, given the type of incentive structure they face, to have a reputation for providing low-quality care? The answer is that to some extent they do, especially with respect to the type of care they provide in cases where patients seek care for relatively minor illnesses. At the same time, US HMOs have to compete with providers that operate on the basis of fee-for-service (and treat patients who are covered by conventional insurance). Given this, the extent to which they

can allow the quality of care to suffer is limited by the fact that if they do they risk losing clients to conventional insurance.

35. In a system of managed care there may be a conflict between the ability of funding agencies to negotiate terms with service providers such as hospitals if care managers also have the right to decide to which providers they will refer their patients. Such a conflict also arises if patients are allowed relatively unrestricted choice of providers. For example, if neither funding agencies nor hospitals can predict the number of patients who will choose to go to any particular hospital for elective surgery, the bargaining situation becomes more complicated, and problems of crowding, on the one hand, and excess capacity, on the other, may arise.

   A catch-phrase used to describe the principle of population-based funding and negotiated contracts is "money should follow the patient" — that is, a provider (within or outside the funding agency's jurisdiction) should be funded in proportion to the services rendered to patients for whom that agency is responsible. From the viewpoint of funding agencies, the task of negotiating contracts would be facilitated if it were possible to make "patients follow the money" — that is, restrict the patient's freedom of choice.

36. The freedom to choose the family doctor is integral to the recent Swedish reforms. However, the attempt to also introduce freedom for patients to choose among hospitals is creating problems.

37. In the US, the Medicare plan offers both these types of choice. On the one hand, enrollees may choose the option of belonging to an HMO, and receive a small premium rebate if they do. On the other hand, while the Medicare plan itself has substantial deductibles, enrollees may elect to purchase supplementary private insurance ("Medigap insurance"), which covers most or all of the Medicare deductibles. For an empirical analysis of the market for such insurance, see J. R. Wolfe and John H. Goddeeris, "Adverse Selection, Moral Hazard, and Wealth Effects in the Medigap Insurance Market," *Journal of Health Economics,* Vol. 10 (1991), pp. 423–50.

   Freedom of choice with respect to insurance is an important element of the original version of the Clinton Plan, under which the funding agencies (referred to as "health alliances") would be obliged to offer at least one fee-for-service plan (in addition to managed care plans), and in which consumers would have an incentive to choose low-cost plans since they would be responsible for a portion of the premium cost. Competition among "care insurers" would also be present in the Dekker proposals for health reform in Holland.

38. For a discussion of these problems, see Blomqvist, *Sound Advice: Prescriptions for Health Care Reform in Canada;* and Blomqvist and Brown (eds.), *Limits to Care.*

39. Although it is not clear in what sense it has been threatened, a stock item in the platforms of several federal parties in recent elections has been to "save Medicare."

M O N I Q U E   J É R Ô M E - F O R G E T

A N D   C L A U D E   E .   F O R G E T

Internal Markets

in the Canadian Context*

The old adage that "if it ain't broke, don't fix it" should be borne in mind by would-be public policy reformers in any domain. In the case of health care reform, the exhortation deserves particular consideration. Canada has a universal system where treatment is based largely on need, and is ranked near the top when it comes to many measures of health status, such as life expectancy.[1] The remarkable level of pride citizens exhibit in the system,[2] due in large part to health care's role as a defining national characteristic distinguishing Canada from its neighbour to the south, also suggests we should be cautious in responding to calls for radical change. All the same, the Canadian health care system is far from perfect. It is not only very costly, but is hampered by an organizational structure under which too little emphasis is placed on the demands of patients.

---

* This paper is a summary of a more developed proposal by the same authors in a forthcoming IRPP monograph.

THE COSTS

While Canada does manage to spend less per capita on health care than the United States, there is little cause for complacency. If the US is left out of per-capita cost comparisons (as it probably should be, given its unique heavy reliance on private market provision), then Canada has far and away the most expensive health care system in the world. Sweden spends only 75 percent as much as Canada, Japan just 66 percent and the United Kingdom a mere 54 percent.[3] If Canada could reduce its expenditure to the level spent by the United Kingdom, the annual savings would amount to almost $31 billion. That's enough money to fund the entire Department of Defence three times over or to eliminate very nearly the annual federal deficit.

There is nothing inherently wrong with spending lots of money on health care. On the contrary, in a publicly funded system, spending levels represent one measure of Canada's desire to establish a relatively equitable society and to respond to a wide range of needs. However, this is only fully true if every extra dollar of expenditure actually results in another dollar's worth of health care provision. This, unfortunately, is not the case. The problem with the current Canadian system is not that so much money is spent, but that so much of total health expenditure is impossible to justify.

Consider, first, some anecdotal evidence. William Weiss, a doctor from Ontario, has pointed out that common aspirin prescribed to senior citizens costs mere pennies per pill, yet for every prescription filled Medicare pays out eight dollars (in addition to the actual cost of the aspirin). He has estimated that asking patients to simply buy aspirin over the counter, even if they are later reimbursed, could save tens of millions of dollars annually.[4]

There are many other examples of specific procedures or failures in co-ordination that lead to increased health care expenditures. Far more pervasive and costly, however, is the persistent tendency for health care costs to increase in general and *en masse*. This is referred to as the "medical-specific" rate of inflation, a measure of the degree to which prices of medical-related goods and services rise faster than the overall consumer price index. In the 30 years between 1960 and 1990, Canada's "real" expenditure on health care rose almost fivefold (or by 493 percent).[5] During those same 30 years, however, the cumulative effect of the fact that health sector prices rose faster than the general level of inflation meant that roughly 33 percent[6] of the extra expenditure was not used to provide more services (x-ray machines, doctors, etc.) but simply to cover inflated costs.

If the expenditure and inflation picture is broken down by decade, some interesting details emerge. Medical-specific inflation was quite high during the 1960s, averaging 1.4 percent per annum. Relating this to the expenditure data allows us to measure the "increase in real health benefits" (or IRHB), which essentially shows how much more *real* health services were provided each year. The IRHB figure for the 1960s averages 4.7 percent per year, demonstrating that, even though medical-specific inflation was quite high, real spending increased much faster. For the 1970s, a decade when even the health care sector had trouble keeping up with overall inflation, the medical-specific measure averaged just 0.3 percent per year. The IRHB average for the same decade was 3.8 percent, and so real provision was growing more slowly than it had a decade earlier. This trend continued through the 1980s, when medical-specific inflation shot up to 1.8 percent and the IRHB fell to 2.5 percent. To put it another way, health care expenditure grew by roughly 10 percent each year throughout the 1980s, yet the real provision of health services grew by only 2.5 percent. Table 1 illustrates this trend.

Some analysts have shrugged this off, assuming that the higher inflation observed in health services in effect reflects increases in the *quality of the inputs* brought about by technological change. This explanation is misleading for a number of reasons. First, the health sector is very labour intensive: technological change embodied in new drugs and medical equipment accounts for only a very small share of total health expenditure. As well, the publicly funded health care system in Canada and Western Europe is the only significant employer of people with health sector-specific skills: as a result, the employer is likely to capture much of any total increase in labour productivity. In addition, technological change does not always push costs up; indeed, such changes have often led to dramatic jumps in efficiency. And even if such efficiency gains translate into higher consumption, this constitutes product-based, not sector-specific, inflation. Finally, health services technology is virtually the same in all western countries and yet health sector-specific inflation varies considerably from country to country.

If the price rises in medical services had been kept in line with over-

Table 1

Health Care Costs, Inflation and Changes in Real Benefits Per Capita

Average annual percentage rates of increase

	1960-70	1970-80	1980-90
Change in Nominal Spending	9.4	12.4	10.2
Medical-Specific Inflation	1.4	0.3	1.8
Increase in Real Health Benefits	4.7	3.8	2.5

SOURCE: OECD, *OECD Health Systems* (Paris: OECD, 1993).

all inflation, the savings would have been enormous. Because this did not happen, $14.1 billion[7] of our expenditures by 1990 had not gone to buy more health provision, but simply to pay more for the health provision we are buying.

How to Protect the Canadian Health System from Inappropriate — Even Fatal — Remedies

The relatively high cost of the Canadian health system is no longer a well-kept secret. Awareness of the trend is particularly widespread among federal and provincial finance department and treasury officials. These agencies of government have for years been closely involved in the analysis of health budgets and major health spending decisions. With the growing realization, in government circles, of the need to reduce deficits and stop the accumulation of public debt, this growing familiarity with health system issues made itself even more acutely felt in the 1990s. All provinces have embarked on belt-tightening measures and some, notably Alberta, have made drastic cuts. For all of that, in spite of economic recovery, the financial situation of governments has not materially improved. As a consequence, the health system is likely to have to bear budget reductions and other measures designed to shrink the total resources devoted to health care.

Provincial governments have taken steps to contain health expenditures, including curbs on wage and fee increases and reduced enrolments in medical schools and reduced numbers of slots available for specialist training. Some hospitals have been closed down by government fiat. Although such measures can create savings, they do not reverse the long-term trend of increasing costs due to greater demand for care and longer life expectancy.

Robert Evans has usefully demonstrated some of the advantages of Canada's health care system over that of the US.[8] One such advantage lies in Canada's single payer system, which is quite unlike the mixed arrangement that prevails in the United States. Yet the strength of this lever for cost control tempts governments to reduce costs while leaving those who manage the system to cope with the consequences.

Over the past 20-odd years, the Canadian system has decentralized responsibility for the consequences of cost control through global budgeting of hospitals. This system has played a very useful role in a period of rapid change in medical technology and modes of practice. Local managers have been able to shift resources as needed with a minimum of red tape, despite working within the context of a publicly funded system. In a complex system with many autonomous institutions, each with its own characteristics, any change brought about by innovation has an uneven impact, giving rise to unevenly distributed windfall gains and losses.[9] This is tolerable in a context where total resources are gently rising for everyone. Once funding is static or starts to decrease, those windfalls become a source of tension. In this process, efficiency gains achieved in some hospitals are hard to translate into savings in others, as budgeters do not want to impose serious budget cuts on the less efficient institutions for fear of a political outcry or of putting them out of business. Strategies such as area or regional agencies are at best experimental attempts to overcome this problem.

Yet, given that only people who actually deliver services can know what services are most appropriate for specific patients, some sort of decentralized global budgeting is advisable. The question is whether current Canadian methods can be improved.

SOME CURRENT CONCEPTS FOR HEALTH CARE RATIONALIZATION

Most diagnostic or therapeutic procedures have never been rigorously evaluated. It is also true that even when they have been, their use in specific circumstances may raise a number of questions about their appropriateness even if only from an ethical perspective. Many studies on the effectiveness of medical procedures are put forward as the basis for rationalizing (read limiting, constraining or rationing) health care by means other than financial.

Some of these efforts — for instance, scientific comparative evaluations of medical technologies or the search for agreed-upon definitions of medical practice — have a significant but, on the whole, modest contribution to make to health care rationalization. Organizations mandated to conduct evaluations of medical technologies have been set up in virtually all developed countries. Their output already constitutes a significant addition to health care literature.

Technology evaluation is useful where there are alternative options and where practitioners have been divided over preferred treatment.

Professional consensus can be achieved out of that disagreement — although this is not an easy task.[10] Often such work has to be updated due to new information (which does not make guidelines in general more credible). Even if planners and managers can be convinced to change their behaviour, getting doctors to change theirs is more difficult.

One popular suggestion is to make sure that physicians are provided with better information on the (cost) effectiveness of various procedures and treatments and then have their decisions reviewed by panels of fellow doctors. This approach has its drawbacks. First, there is the obvious increase in the demand on a doctor's time. As well, such panels would inevitably interfere with the important right of doctors to choose what they feel is the most appropriate treatment for their patients. This sort of bureaucratic attempt to force alternatives on physicians is likely to increase resentment, exacerbate the problem of lack of responsiveness to patients and have only a negligible effect on expenditures.[11]

An even more questionable approach consists of attempts to identify a social or political consensus on "basic services" for funding purposes, from either a public or private (i.e., insurance) perspective. The "Oregon Experiment," an effort to turn this concept into an operational plan, has attracted much publicity. Although the state of Oregon, with the federal government's approval, began to implement the plan in 1994, doubts remain with regard to conceptual flaws. Even with a few hundred "treatment-condition" pairs, such a plan constitutes a very severe abstraction from a much more complex reality. As a result, its very credibility may rapidly suffer in the eyes of physicians first and the general public thereafter. This is likely to lead to efforts to circumvent the restrictions the plan imposes, thereby nullifying its effect. Plans such as this are clearly not applicable in Canada or any other country committed to universal coverage and a single-tier system: Oregon-type limitations could only affect insurability, not the provision of health care, and therefore — and in the name of equity! — they would automatically result in a two-tier system.[12]

Given the almost infinite number of combinations of pathologies, medical conditions, individual preferences, professional skills, family circumstances and ethical views, any attempt to find recipes with general applicability is doomed. In a totally privatized and uninsured context, the patient-physician relationship is where all those factors would be reconciled, presumably in an optimal way. This "ideal" — if indeed it is one — is unattainable for several reasons. The best system arguably is one that approximates the situation of reciprocal, informed interaction between physician and patient.

Given both the need sometimes to finance very expensive procedures and to do so through a feasible and reasonable use of resources, the formula that imposes the fewest outside constraints on physician-patient interaction remains one in which a "single payer" determines budgets but in which resources are allocated in a highly decentralized process built around the patient-physician relationship.

THE HEALTH SERVICES SECTOR: NOT A MONOLITH

All the current approaches by which proponents seek to introduce internal market arrangements share the same basic and important assumption about the health services sector — that it is *not* a monolithic structure. For at least 30 years, discussions about health care have been dominated, especially in Canada, by the planner's perspective. This has been predicated on the fact that health services are (in most western countries) a segment of the public sector, making it appear natural to look at health services systems as single entities.

The health care sector, however, is no more monolithic than the financial sector, the telecommunications industry or any other economic grouping where thousands of firms compete and interact, buying and selling services from and to one another. In each of these areas, there are raw material suppliers, manufacturers, wholesalers, retailers, large and small firms, niche players specializing in certain products or providing specialized services to other firms, etc.

The health services sector exhibits similar diversity. While in most industries the many participants interact through markets, in the health sector, with only a few exceptions, the interactions among the different parts have been governed by a system of command and control. Money and prices play a far less important role, since each interacting part is funded by the government, either directly or through some other central public agency.

Whatever the implicit assumptions behind the command-and-control system, reality has been seen to conflict with the blissful image of organizations such as not-for-profit hospitals spontaneously pursuing the public good. This reality has first led to a search for political remedies designed to enhance the accountability of the health care institutions to the public: the election of members of regional or district boards or hospital boards or requirements that such boards were to report to elected public institutions in order to provide discipline. These organizations, despite the undoubted goodwill on which they draw, have disappointed because they have been powerless to shift their attention from the aspirations of providers to the expectations of clients.

CREATING A "MARKET" AND DEVISING AN EFFECTIVE AGENT

The following discussion simply takes for granted that patients, i.e., customers of the health services industry, need an "agent" to purchase services on their behalf.[13]

The two concepts "agents" and "internal markets" are important and complementary. Starting from a vision of the health services industry as a large, complex and diversified set of interrelated but distinct activities, our proposal provides a way to organize these interrelationships based on a quasi-market model. The markets are *internal* because they involve, on both the demand and supply sides, entities from within the publicly funded health sector itself. This concept can be contrasted with *external* markets, where at least one of the participants (buyer or seller) is outside the health sector. Examples of outside participants that interact with the health sector are electricity utilities, food suppliers, individuals selling their own labour, etc.

Fundamental to internal markets is the idea that in each market there would be, on one side of the transaction, a "purchaser" organization that is an integral part of the health services sector itself but that operates as the patient's agent. On the selling side, there would be another health services entity.

The search for an effective agent (to act as a purchaser on behalf of patients) has led different countries along different paths. The resulting arrangements are discussed in several papers in this volume. Drawing inspiration from them, and from other considerations sometimes overlooked in the existing institutions, this paper proposes a quasi-market organization of health services that has as its central focus what might be called a Targeted Medical Agency (TMA).

Physicians as Agents

The overriding purpose of the arrangements presented here is to focus more effectively on patients' requirements in terms of effectiveness and quality of care. Physicians, more than any other constituent part of the health care system, have been trained (witness the "Hippocratic Oath") with this type of concern in mind. Any reorganization of the health services system should strengthen this already significant element. As in the British GP fundholding approach, our proposal seeks to build upon physician professionalism. Therefore, we propose giving physicians the patient agency role.

Other quasi-market structures give the patient agency role to bureaucratic organizations. Regional health authorities, private insurers or even HMOs with hundreds of thousands of clients are primarily bureaucratic structures whose managers attempt to evaluate and control physicians' activities and decisions. This results in a hierarchical chain of command over the professional activity of physicians. The universal experience with those efforts is that they work very imperfectly, if at all.

Success would be defined as a combination of greater overall efficiency (i.e., more output for the same input, or the same output for less input) combined with resulting administrative costs that would not exceed the efficiency savings inherent in the promise of internal markets.[14] British District Health Authorities may have been able to contain overall cost increases by relying on global budgets, but do not seem to have increased the throughput of the system through efficiency gains. American insurers may have generated strong incentives to keep some input costs down, but at high administrative cost and with large increases in overall spending. HMOs initially had much success in improving efficiency, mostly by reducing recourse to hospitals, but were no better than insurers at capping overall cost increases.

In order to prevent the bureaucratization that would inevitably set in, there should be a ceiling on the number of physicians who could band together to form a TMA; while any number must be arbitrary, 25 or 30 seems a defensible maximum number, with an average figure considerably less.

Some may argue that the market could decide any "ceiling" on the size of TMAs based on physicians' and patients' preferences. This is a seductive argument. The danger to guard against, however, arises from the expected physician response to the novelty of the concept: namely to entrust the formation of the first TMAs to *entrepreneurs* less intimidated by change than physicians themselves. This could quickly bring about the formation of very large TMAs, which might establish a position of dominance, leaving physicians and patients with no effective choice. In addition, maintaining *choice* for patients among a number of TMAs requires the existence of relatively small and numerous TMAs in most regions.

TMAs constitute a scheme that, contrary to the British fundholding formula, would not be restricted to general practitioners. In North America (and this holds for Canada) there is no tradition of general practitioners acting as gatekeepers. Patients have traditionally self-referred themselves to specialists in private practice or, increasingly, in hospital outpatient clinics. The gatekeeper function by one class of physicians over the entire system, although attractive enough to have inspired many health planners' dreams and several aborted initiatives, is sociologically unpalatable.

In any case, specialists have, in reality, an even greater impact on the use of resources in the health services sector than general practitioners do. As will presently be explained, the arrangements we propose give them a different role from that of general practitioners but fully recognize their potential contribution as patients' agents.

Patients will be able to move between TMAs as their preferences and evolving medical conditions dictate. This ability will maintain much of the patient choice that is inherent in the existing system. Those services that TMAs purchase from other suppliers, such as outside treatments, diagnostics and the like, will be the only options that are constrained from the patient's perspective under this system. This issue of choice has emerged as a fundamental point in current American debates on health care reform, and is therefore important to consider. Some restriction on choice is necessary; in order for medical decisions to be made in efficient, cost-conscious ways, there must be a single agent who bears responsibility for the financial consequences of these choices. This proposal preserves the right of patients to choose their main source of care and to alter that choice by switching to another TMA, but does not allow for full patient choice of supplier for each individual procedure or treatment within a given TMA. The loss of choice will certainly be more than compensated for by the overall transition of the system to a greatly more patient-centred mode of organization.

Comprehensive Payment by Capitation

Our proposal is embedded in the current Canadian (and dominant West European) financing model for health services: universal income-related fiscal levy. Suggested changes concern only how the resulting fund is *disbursed*, not how it is *raised*. The existing Canadian practice of global budget financing should also be maintained, since it is a practice that has been relatively successful in controlling hospital costs. Beyond that point, the required changes are radical.

At present, in Canada, hospitals are funded by global budgets, but physicians are paid, by and large, by fee-for-service (FFS). We propose a 180° shift; physicians would operate under a budget and hospitals would be financed in large part through FFS. However, since hospital services would be requested and paid for by TMAs out of their own "budgets," our proposal in effect would extend to the *whole* of the health care sector the restraints of global budgeting, while putting physicians in charge of budget allocation among different services. This would include not only their own services, but also hospital-based diagnostic procedures and hospital-based "infrastructure" equipment and services.

The "budgets" with which physicians (grouped within TMAs) would operate would result from aggregating annual capitation payments. From the patient's point of view, this is a voucher system, a financial credit instrument that follows the patient wherever he chooses to go to obtain a comprehensive bundle of services for a given period of time. It is a payment for a contract between the patient and the TMA, where the latter accepts responsibility to provide to the patient, by itself or by out-sourcing, *any* health service required to maintain and/or restore that patient's health for that period of time.

In all classes of TMAs, physicians stand to benefit substantially from these proposed reforms. They would have control over how resources are spent in a way that can only be achieved by an agent holding the purse strings. If doctors are frustrated by slow service from diagnostics, or hear complaints from patients about treatment at referral sites, they have the financial authority to take their business elsewhere. This empowerment serves the dual roles of bringing the patients' needs closer to decision makers and also generating downward pressure on prices. There are already indications from the UK that the first of these objectives can be achieved by employing internal market forms of organization that keep the size of the purchasing body relatively small and non-bureaucratic.[15]

Doctor control over the demand side of resource allocation is also in harmony with the ethical training of physicians.

Targeted Financing and Organization of Physicians' Agencies

As a number of other authors in this volume have shown, any system in which lump sums are paid for either insurance or health services is subject to exploitation in the form of "risk selection" or "cream skimming."[16] We believe these concerns are not as critical as some suggest, for several reasons.

First, the literature on variations in the use of resources among countries or regions where there is little concomitant variation in health outcomes suggests that there is room for a more conservative use of health services. Unless cream skimming creates huge disparities in the risk profiles of different TMAs' groups of patients, any group of physicians should be able to meet reasonable expense targets while still maintaining high-quality care.

Second, while it is true that any recipient of funds will seek to use factors that are not considered in a risk-adjustment formula in order to cream skim, it is also true that, when such measures are found, the government is likely to discover them as well, and in short order. It will then add them to the formula. In short, the process of risk selection and risk adjustment is iterative, and the government is unlikely to fall too far behind. Indeed, over time any exploiters of the system are likely to run out of new measures.

Third, a major source of cream skimming could be knowledge of prior medical conditions.[17] Supporters of traditional internal market proposals have trouble addressing differences among patients with these conditions because they assume that plans should have similar treatment capacities. Our TMA proposal reverses that logic: instead of seeking to create systems with similar capacities to treat everyone the same, we encourage differentiation.

Several studies have shown that strong incentives for cream skimming arise if "prior medical condition" is not part of the capitation formula.[18] Patients with, for instance, a critical heart condition, or suffering from diabetes, require substantially more resources than patients with a "clean record." There are powerful financial incentives inherent in a uniform capitation payment to encourage doctors to attempt to send patients with heavier demands for health care elsewhere. Similarly, the windfall gains to be had for those doctors treating a lower number of such more demanding clients are also large, and would needlessly inflate system costs. Taking account of all of these determining factors in establishing a capitation formula can, however, lead to other problems, such as creating incentives for TMAs to dishonestly classify patients into high-paying groups.

The key would be to develop a set of different capitation prices for different conditions, such as diabetes or heart problems. Then TMAs that specialized in care for such conditions would be likely to treat them more efficiently (and successfully) than other providers, so would have both economic and professional incentives to seek those patients.

What is clear from the ongoing Dutch experience,[19] and from the British difficulties[20] in establishing formula-based funding, is that capitation arrangements are not a trivial hurdle. There is, however, no reason to believe that producing an effective form of payment is impossible. A variety of proposals for dealing with this problem exists[21] and, though there is much work and research to be done, the final fall-back position is that there is no need for the capitation formula to be carved in stone. As long as it is malleable on reasonably short notice, any significant problems, such as systematic TMA avoidance of a given payment class (which might require some sort of monitoring), can be addressed as they occur by changing the magnitude of the payment.

The obvious need to reflect in a differentiated level of capitation payments not only the age and sex but also prior medical conditions suggests, at the same time, the need to have medical agencies that are targeted at the range of special requirements.

For instance, community-oriented, primary care TMAs composed essentially of general practitioners could naturally target patients with clean medical records who form the single largest group of patients. On the other hand, hospital-based, secondary and tertiary care TMAs composed essentially of physicians with a related cluster of sub-specialties would also naturally target clients with one or a few prior medical conditions. The potential also exists for mixed TMAs where primary and secondary care doctors might join together in order to satisfy some group of patient demands. The essential features are only that they be relatively small (to ensure competition among them) and that they be the purchasers of all of the health services their patients require.

The specialist-based TMAs envisaged here are not entire hospitals any more than they are traditional hospital departments. Why not? If hospitals, lock, stock and barrel, were to become TMAs, they would, by definition, fail one of the tests for a successful reform already described: they would be bureaucratic structures attempting to play the role of patients' agents. There is no guarantee that their effectiveness in this role would be adequate, because the TMAs with that structure would not be able to overcome the perennial handicap of hospital management — namely, the duality of their leadership, with management on one side and physicians on the other.

A Two-Envelope System

We propose here a comprehensive capitation payment system resulting in a global budget for each TMA that corresponds to its client base. Funds would be allocated to pay not only for services provided by the professional partners making up the TMA (mostly but not necessarily comprised of physicians), but also for purchasing from other TMAs, community organizations or hospitals the complementary services needed by their clients.

The determination of capitation payments is not discussed in this short paper. However, we can observe that establishing the payments is not a major problem, given the single payer situation that prevails in Canada. Utilization profiles reflecting age, sex and even area of residence are already known. The impact of a prior medical condition or some other factors could also be estimated on the basis of the utilization data for medical acts and the related payments made to professionals for each individual. Finally an iterative process, based on annual or more frequent revisions could introduce a progressive refinement in capitation rates. All the data required for such calculations are more readily available in Canada than in most other countries.

The sums making up the TMA's budget would consist of two envelopes. The first, the remuneration pool, would be destined to pay for the partners' own remuneration; the other and larger one — held as it were as a trust — would finance purchases from the rest of the system. This trust fund is what would empower TMAs to become effective buyers of services on behalf of patients. Faced with the limitations of this (risk-weighted) budget, they would be made conscious of the need to choose treatment and other forms of care that are cost-effective. This trust envelope would need to be adequate to purchase not only narrowly defined medical and hospital services, but also all community-based services including follow-up care, purchased from GP-based TMAs, home care, etc.

All the diagnostic services (x-rays, blood tests, etc.) required would be purchased in the same way or generated internally if that is more efficient. If performed internally, these services would, however, have to be funded from the procuring envelope. These services do not directly benefit patients, but are only useful to generate data that guide medical decision making: in the economists' jargon, they are "intermediate goods." A case could be made to share that cost between the trust fund and the remuneration pool (once that pool had been adjusted accordingly) so as to introduce a strong incentive for a more judicious use of all the rapidly burgeoning data-generation activity. This would also help limit the effects of expensive "gee-whiz" technology purchases on the system's overall costs, since any diagnostic service purchase would be the result of a decision by a physician with an eye to cost-effectiveness. If a standard x-ray or physical exam can reveal the problem, there is no need to use expensive Magnetic Resonance Imaging scanners.

Similarly, one could envisage an efficiency-motivated reduction in capitation payments phased in over a number of years. That planned reduction would translate into a phased reduction in the trust funds managed by TMAs. The TMAs could be given a financial incentive to achieve planned reductions in the form of a fraction of the savings being transferred to the remuneration pool. However, as previous discussions along these lines have indicated, the very possibility that such measures may give the appearance that physicians can make a "profit" by restricting access to services might arouse strong emotional reactions among the public. Given that our proposal would apply within the context of a publicly funded system, this notion needs to be considered carefully.

However, such an approach may be made easier in light of the need to provide for a corresponding penalty. For instance, assume that a particular TMA has exhausted its trust fund for the year at the end of the tenth month, leaving a two-month deficiency in funds needed to pay for services bought on behalf of its clients. How would this be made up? How, more generally, would "overspending" be discouraged? The central concept lies in affirming the TMA's responsibility for living within its overall capitation-based budget; hence the TMA would borrow against future remuneration pool payments if the shortfall is too large to be absorbed by the current-year remuneration pool.

This proposal does not involve the concept of "core services" or any procedure to define such a concept. Efforts to turn the notion of "essential health services" into an operational definition inevitably get bogged down in bureaucratizing health care or, eventually, turning the whole issue over to the courts — which comes to the same thing. The notion of "core services" is a plausible outcome of the competitive system envisaged in this paper and it would be given several definitions — not just one — in this context.

A Multiplicity of Internal Markets

Because our proposed system is centred on clients rather than on a specific class of providers, it would result in a multiplicity of internal markets for a great variety of services, each involving several potential purchasers and vendors: not only between TMAs and hospitals but between TMAs and community resources and between TMAs and other TMAs.

This is distinct from the British fundholding concept, which reserves for GPs the role of purchasers and restricts other players to the role of vendors. In our proposed scheme, specialist-based TMAs may purchase follow-up care from GP-based TMAs. The latter may purchase from the former special diagnostic expertise for their clients. It is even more important for specialist-based TMAs to have access to, and funds to purchase services from, low-cost, community-based organizations to avoid leaving patients with serious medical conditions in the high-cost, not very user-friendly, specialized care echelon. Finally, the small size of the typical TMA ensures that all of these internal markets exhibit a substantial degree of competition. This is an essential point. Quality of care at an acceptable cost cannot be achieved with organizations whose large size would pre-empt the entire local or regional market. Large size is bad by itself if it interferes with the personal, direct bond between physician and patient, but it has the further defect of making impossible an effective choice among agencies.

Small groupings are also required in order to attack one of the major problems with the current system: persistent medical-specific inflation. By forcing TMAs to compete with one another to supply services and, more importantly, by placing purchasing decisions in the hands of ground-level physicians within TMAs, this set of proposals would generate cost-consciousness on the demand side of the market. Aware of their duty to provide care, and of the financial repercussions of losing patients, physicians will naturally seek out cost-effective treatments to buy on behalf of their patients. The ability to buy diagnostics, such as x-ray services, from a number of competing suppliers will certainly exert downward pressure on prices.

Would so many market transactions make the system unwieldy by increasing information costs beyond reason? That is a significant issue that will need to be answered in greater detail. Let us note, however, that the small scale of TMAs, where members have the status of partners, will mean that informal processes typical of small business will be used rather than highly formalized public tendering procedures. Most transactions will be repetitive and therefore use the same information base.

Client Registration and Hand-Off

In this discussion we have so far avoided the question of how clients and targeted medical agencies would pair off. As well, patients with clean medical records would evolve over time into patients with pre-existing medical conditions; how could the transfer or "hand-off" between a GP-based TMA and a specialist-based TMA take place? In analyzing these issues, we have to remain aware of possible dysfunctional incentives to gain an illegitimate advantage for either client or agency.

The pairing off of clean-record clients and GP-based TMAs seems relatively problem-free. Clients with significant prior medical conditions, if properly informed about the system, have little reason to apply to such an agency and the agency has no incentive to take them on as they are by definition high-cost clients. For clean-record patients, the pairing off might therefore take place on the basis of proximity, word-of-mouth, favourable publicity, cultural affinity in multicultural communities, etc. It is likely that TMAs would actively solicit clients, since each new registrant would bring an additional capitation payment. One can imagine an interest to segment the "clean-record market" so to speak. "Well mother and baby" TMAs (probably with a specific capitation level) or geriatric or women's TMAs (probably also with a specific capitation level) would not offend anyone's sense of propriety, and would be consistent with a client focus.

The higher-cost "prior medical condition" markets pose more difficult but not insurmountable problems. What one has to guard against here is self-appointment by essentially clean-record clients to more expensive, specialist-based TMAs, along with a spurious but mutually beneficial prior medical condition triggering a higher capitation payment.

As a rule, the freedom of clients to change from one TMA to another should be unfettered. This freedom is the only workable means of making client preferences for a style of service delivery effective. Changes of residence or changes in medical status could trigger shifts in client registrations with TMAs. With capitation being paid for comprehensive coverage over a period of time, rather than for specific procedures, pre-notification would probably be needed either a month or a quarter in advance, depending on how payments were made. Would every person have to register? As an income-related levy would be collected from everyone, non-registration would cause a fund to accumulate that could presumably be used to pay for services on a fee-for-service basis up to an amount equal to each person's applicable, differentiated capitation rate; anything above that could be at the client's expense.

This *laissez-faire* attitude toward the possibility of non-registration may alarm some readers as opening the door to a two-tiered system. It is mentioned here mostly as a way to ease transitional difficulties between the two systems. However, the proposal must also be understood against the background of the current Canadian financial system, where private insurance is ruled out. Hence, the potential penalty for non-registration will be a very sizeable cost to the individual non-registrant since the capitation fee level, when used as a ceiling for reimbursements, will only cover a small part of the costs associated with serious illness. As well, at least at the beginning, non-registration would be the rule rather than the exception as too few TMAs would exist. Therefore, reimbursements would have to be topped up, perhaps through a scale of payments established to decline to the capitation level ceiling once the new system was fully in place.

This generally free-choice setting provides the backdrop against which we must resolve the question of how a patient can "graduate" from a low-cost capitation category to a higher-cost one. With age-differentiated capitation rates, the graduation would be automatic. Patients in need of one-time specialist services, such as an appendectomy, would certainly stay with their regular TMA and have this procedure purchased for them. The remaining class of individuals who have to graduate to a higher-cost medical status must be addressed carefully. A three-corner process suggests itself. First, the patient needs to be informed about his evolving medical condition, recognize a need for transfer and approve the selection of the specialist-based TMA of destination. Second, the TMA of origin, by definition, would have been responsible for carrying out the evaluation of a client's medical condition that led to the requirement of a transfer and would have to agree to it as representing its best advice to that patient. This is different from the British GP's gatekeeper role in one important respect. If the transfer occurs, the TMA of origin would lose forever the capitation that accompanies that patient, but would also cease to be professionally and financially responsible for her or him. If the transfer is "premature," as compared to an objective needs assessment, the TMA may lose control over more revenues than those needed to continue to look after that client.

This incentive not to transfer prematurely may not, however, be sufficient to counteract the opposite incentive by the receiving TMA to prematurely "acquire" a client with below-average needs to join the ranks of a higher-cost group of clients.

For reasons such as these, proposals incorporating capitation payments have sometimes included incentive schemes in the form of a target bonus payable to primary care TMAs for keeping their "clean-record patients" in that status (i.e., in good health), coupled with a reduction in that target bonus for each client (possibly over an actuarially determined threshold) migrating to a higher-cost category. This is certainly a sensible arrangement.

Further research and discussions are needed to determine whether patients transferred to specialist-based TMAs, along with the correspondingly higher capitation payments, would remain in that situation forever. Data on the cost implications of prior medical conditions are not sufficient at present to allow us to gauge the resulting cost over a number of years. Once a given medical condition has been remedied, or at least stabilized, could not a case be made for returning the follow-up care to a primary care-type TMA? Should targets not be set with this result in mind? It seems reasonable to allow a mechanism to ratchet down capitation payments just as there is one readily imaginable to ratchet them up. This is one area where the authors found the available data and literature to be insufficient to support any generalization. It represents a substantial issue with regard to the effectiveness of medical care, and one that appears quite important to elucidate.

Continuity of Service and Solvency

There are public policy reasons for imposing a ceiling on the size of TMAs: to prevent their bureaucratization and to encourage a competitive environment even in a sparsely populated region. However, there are countervailing pressures. In order to provide continuity of service while ensuring reasonable quality of life for physicians and some expense sharing, group practice has gained in favour. Single-physician TMAs do not appear desirable or likely. Four- or five-physician TMAs seem to represent the smallest viable unit.

However, the obligation to fund a comprehensive range of services, including some very high-cost procedures with very low incidence, is bound to create pressure for large-size TMAs on the basis of spreading those risks over a larger base. Our proposal to have differentiated capitation rates for target groups of clients is bound to reduce considerably the strength of this argument. The British approach to resolving this problem is to cap the cost of procedures that must be funded by the fundholders. The current British limit is set at £5,000. This, in effect, is akin to a reinsurance "stop-loss" policy. Another approach is to allow TMAs to build up financial reserves for unusual deviations, a piece of financial management that TMAs may find difficult to perform themselves and that could, therefore, be contracted out to financial institutions. Government-sponsored schemes to shoulder high-cost procedures or insure TMAs should be resisted as they are bound to introduce confusion as to the real nature of the new structure for managing health services and, over time, encourage a drifting back to the old command-and-control system.

Another approach, inspired from Dutch practice, would consist in allowing each TMA to designate a maximum of two percent of its client base for whom ongoing and anticipated costs exceed the capitation rate by a given stated multiple.[22] Those costs would then be absorbed by some sort of central compensation fund.

The system thus far gives strong incentives to physicians to act as effective agents on behalf of their patients. This framework, however, must be backed up with legitimate penalties for failure to treat patients in a cost-effective manner. The reward for cost savings (i.e., partial trust pool transfers to remuneration pools) requires a corresponding penalty. For example, a trust fund shortfall would have to be made up from the remuneration pool, presumably through a loan repayable over possibly more than one year. TMAs that find themselves insolvent would certainly be required to disband. Beyond that basic threat, several possibilities suggest themselves. One requirement for the formation of a TMA would be equity contributions on the part of its members. If the TMA should fail, that equity would be forfeited. This potential loss would provide strong incentives for member physicians to practise cost-effective medicine. Exact details on exit rules, like most aspects of our proposal, would have to be fully developed in consultation with physicians.

CONCLUSION

The foregoing proposal is inspired by the desire to bank on the known strengths of the existing Canadian system in order to regulate the operations and the interactions of the many and different entities that make up the health services sector. These strengths reside first in the *value system* that shapes physicians' behaviour. That value system incorporates strong, self-confident professionalism — rigorous training that in a manner of speaking "programs" individual practitioners along predictable paths and makes them intolerant of any hierarchical oversight, especially by others than their peers. In this way, professionals share many traits with *entrepreneurs*. That value system also incorporates an ethical view of the relationship of doctor to patient.

Another source of strength lies in the use of *budgets* to circumscribe the area left to the discretion of professionals. Thus budgets help define a minimalist, non-bureaucratic relationship between the health system seen as a whole from a macroeconomic (i.e., financial) perspective and the health system as an operational, day-to-day microeconomic set of innumerable relationships and concrete decisions.

At the same time, we have tried in this proposal to avoid the traps into which so many health services organizations and financing systems have fallen. The first and most important is the *bureaucratic impulse,* to which both US private insurers and many, very different publicly funded systems have fallen prey. The second is the lack of attention to the tendency of any health system to develop above-average *inflation*. Health planners apparently oblivious to the inherent monopolistic and moral hazard features of the medical profession have often added measures that merely reinforced the "cost-plus" reflexes already present. Competition has long been recognized as one of the surest means of achieving cost control.

1. OECD, *OECD Health Systems - The Socio-economic Environment Statistical References* (Paris: OECD, 1993). Based on Statistics Canada, *Life Tables: Canada and Provinces* (Ottawa, 1988); calculated for the three-year period centred around each population census.
2. Robert G. Evans, Morris L. Barer and Clyde Hertzman, "The 20-Year Experiment: Accounting for, Explaining, and Evaluating Health Care Cost Containment in Canada and the United States," *Annual Review of Public Health*, Vol. 12 (1991), pp. 481-518.
3. OECD, *OECD Health Systems - The Socio-economic Environment*, table A2.1.2, p. 67.
4. William Weiss, *Health Care: Conflicting Opinions, Tough Decisions* (Toronto: NC Press Limited, 1992).
5. The rate of increase in real health expenditure (493 percent) was calculated as follows:

    Health expenditure in current dollars totalled 2.142 billion for 1960, and 62.706 billion for 1990. [See *OECD Health Systems - Facts and Trends* (Paris: OECD, 1993), table 4.1.1: Total Expenditure on Health.] To obtain the increase in expenditure in real terms (i.e., without inflation), constant dollars are used. The total expenditure is thus multiplied by the GDP deflator for the year concerned: 2.142* 100/24.7 for 1960, and 62.706* 100/121.4 for 1990. This gives, in constant 1985 dollars, a total expenditure of 8.7 billion for 1960, and 51.6 billion for 1990. (See *OECD Health Systems - The Socio-economic Environment*, table A1.2.4: Price Indices for Gross Domestic Product.) The increase is then (51.6 - 8.7) / 8.7* 100, which is 493 percent.
6. The specific medical inflation accounts for 33 percent of the health expenditure increase. Such proportion was obtained as follows:

    We figured the difference between the growth rate of the medical price index (see *OECD Health Systems - Facts and Trends*, table 4.4.1: Medical Price Index) and the growth rate of the price index for gross domestic product during that period (see *OECD Health Systems - The Socio-economic Environment*, table A1.2.4: Price Indices for Gross

Domestic Product). From 1960 to 1990, Canada's health expenditure in real terms (1985 dollars) jumped from $8.7 billion to $51.6 billion — an increase of $42.9 billion. However, if each year's spending increase were adjusted by assuming that the excess increase from specific medical inflation had not occurred, then the spending at the end of 30 years would have been $14.1 billion less in 1985 dollars. In other words, had the specific medical inflation been zero, health expenditure would have increased from $8.7 billion in 1960 to $37.5 billion in 1990 — an increase of $28.8 billion. Thus, we would have spent $14.1 billion less than we did while still receiving the same amount of services. In other words, 33 percent of the increase of Canada's health expenditure (that is 14.1/42.9), was generated by specific medical inflation.

7.   See OECD publications cited in note 6.

8.   See Evans *et al.*, "The 20-Year Experiment."

9.   The Quebec "Conseil d'évaluation des technologies médicales" has illustrated the way lithotripsy in some tertiary care hospitals has lowered the average cost of kidney stones removals but has led to increased utilization and therefore to resulting cost increases in those hospitals performing the new procedures roughly matched by savings in a large number of referring hospitals. *The Impact of Renal Extracorporeal Shock-Wave Lithotripsy on the Use of Resources in the Quebec Health Care System* (Conseil d'évaluation des technologies de la santé du Québec, June 15, 1994, Montreal).

10.   M. McGregor, "Can Our Health Services Be Saved by Technology Evaluation? The Quebec Experience," Clinical and Investigative Medicine, Vol. 17, no. 4 (1994), pp. 334-42.

11.   Devidas Menon and Sharon Sommerhalder, *Influence of Educational Interventions on the Test Ordering Patterns of Physicians* (Canadian Coordinating Office for Health Technology Assessment, November 1992).

12.   Claude E. Forget, "Who Will Define What Are Essential Health Services?", address delivered as part of the scientific program of the celebration of the Centennial of the Royal Victoria Hospital (Montreal: June 9, 1994). For a strong defense of two-tiered health systems, see H. Tristram Engelhardt, Jr., "Why a Two-Tier System of

Health Care Delivery is Morally Unavoidable," in Martin A. Strosberg, Joshua M. Wiener, Robert Baker, with I. Alan Fein (eds.), *Rationing America's Medical Care: The Oregon Plan and Beyond* (Washington, DC: The Brookings Institution, 1992), pp. 196-207.

13. There is abundant literature on the asymmetry of information with regard to health services that makes it imperative for health services customers (principals) to have recourse to an agent in order to have effective access to those services. The literature on the "principal-agent" problem is pertinent for the present discussion but will not be summarized here. For a comprehensive review, see P. Newman, M. Milgate and John Eatwell (eds.), *The New Palgrave Dictionary of Money and Finance* (Toronto: Macmillan, 1992).

14. See Howard Glennerster, "Internal Markets: Context and Structure," pp. 17-25 in this volume.

15. See Howard Glennester, "Internal Markets: Context and Structure," pp. 17-25 in this volume.

16. See Vivian Hamilton, "Risk Selection: A Major Issue in Internal Markets," pp. 155-64 and Wynand P.M.M van de Ven and Frederik T. Schut, "The Dutch Experience with Internal Markets," pp. 95-117 both in this volume.

17. See, for instance, Howard Glennerster, "Internal Markets: Context and Structure," pp. 17-25 in this volume or W.P.M.M. van de Ven and R.C.J.A. van Vliet, "How can we prevent cream skimming in a competitive health insurance market?", paper presented at The Second World Congress on Health Economics, Zürich, September 10-14, 1990.

18. See Vivian Hamilton, "Risk Selection: A Major Issue in Internal Markets," pp. 155-64 in this volume or Howard Glennerster and Manos Matsaganis, "The Threat of Cream Skimming in the Post-Reform NHS," *Journal of Health Economics*, Vol. 13, no. 1 (March 1994), pp. 31-60.

19. See Wynand P.M.M. van de Ven and Frederik T. Schut, "The Dutch Experience with Internal Markets," pp. 95-117 in this volume.

20. See Howard Glennerster, Manos Matsaganis and Patricia Owens, *Wild Card or Winning Hand?: Implementing Fundholding* (London: London School of Economics, 1993).

21. See Vivian Hamilton, "Risk Selection: A Major Issue in Internal Markets," pp. 155-64 in this volume.
22. See Wynand P.M.M. van de Ven and Frederik T. Schut, "The Dutch Experience with Internal Markets," pp. 95-117 in this volume.

R O B E R T   G .   E V A N S

MANAGING HEALTH CARE REFORM

IN CANADA

INTERNAL MARKETS: GETTING THE TARGETS AND INCENTIVES RIGHT

The fiscal constraints that face Canada as a whole have already had a substantial impact on health care funding. That reality is unlikely to change in the near future, so the question of health care reform becomes one of trying to figure out how to do more with less. Cost-control methods that worked in the past, such as bed closures, must be applied much more tightly in the present environment. Our present circumstance necessarily creates political conflict, which in turn leads to greater interest in new mechanisms and modes of management. It is for precisely these reasons that internal markets are being discussed in Canada.

The complicating issue concerning internal markets is that designing actual systems with effective incentives is an immense task. The choice of incentive — at whom and how it is targeted — is absolutely crucial and is not automatically discernible in any given health context. Many economists would argue that drug expenditures could be reduced if patients had to pay these costs themselves. The reality is that drugs are not a consumption good. They are an input in the production of good health. If consumers are forced to pay separately for a particular production input, it is not very surprising that producers will tend to over-use it. The importance of this example is that any incentive-based reforms have to be carefully thought out, rather than implemented as knee-jerk responses to increasing costs.

Two more examples illustrate my point. It has recently come to light that new policies in Quebec for increasing organ donations have met with some measure of success. The process that Quebec is now following is essentially one of paying bounties to hospitals for success. The standard rhetoric from economists is that if organ donations are lower than desired, then paying donors will solve the problem. In this case, at least, the economists were wrong. The lesson is that one can use the market, or market-like incentives, with considerable success if one is very careful to target who it is that should react.

Another example comes from Germany, where the reimbursement rules for physicians' prescriptions for pharmaceuticals were recently altered. The new regulations require that if payments exceed firm targets the excess is taken from the budget available for reimbursing physicians. Within the first six months there was an almost 20-percent drop in pharmaceutical claims. The Germans found the right target and gave it the right incentives. This approach stands in stark contrast to the Canadian response of suggesting that co-payments be increased, which is another market-like proposal but one that simply does not work.

INTERNAL MARKETS IN CANADA

The Canadian health care system could be characterized as already employing internal markets, at least relative to Nordic Countries, because it separates the provider and the payer. It is not clear how tight that separation is when provincial governments can replace all the members of a hospital board, or the management, or the doctors, or the janitor. But Canada does have an internal market in the sense that, for physicians at least, money follows the patient. So long as there is a large supply of doctors in this country, as there is, they tend to be very glad to see patients, particularly in primary care. They may not want to see them for very long, but the general willingness is there.

Another peculiar sort of internal market is created in the conflict between fee-for-service physicians and budgeted hospitals. There is a reliance on physicians to exert pressure on hospitals to increase throughput when capacity is reduced. Historically, this has been successful; the throughput of Canadian hospitals has been going steadily up while bed supply has been going steadily down. The economic interests of physicians are thus juxtaposed with the economic incentives of hospitals. The standard criticism from the United States that Canada has an inefficient "public utility" health care system is simply unfounded.

In Canada there is a risk that, rather than looking at internal markets, we will be diverted by what I would call "parallel" or "marginal" markets. Parallel markets are the attempt to develop private systems alongside a public one, the purpose being to keep the overall system expanding. This allows the costs to keep growing, because every dollar of cost is a dollar of someone's income. This means that the rhetoric of markets and market mechanisms can be used to try to avoid any kind of improvement in efficiency in the existing system, and, rather, to find off-budget ways of expanding it.

The same is true of what might be called marginal markets, whereby extra charges are imposed on those who are able to pay. The point, again, is to make more money flow through the system, rather than less. This stands in contrast to a true internal market, which is one that tries to operate under a global constraint and actually change the efficiency and effectiveness of the existing system.

More Management, Not More Money

Internal markets are best thought of as a management tool: something that the Canadian system may be turning toward because growing expenditures are out-pacing the ability of the old cost-containment schemes to work. Management must work at three different levels. First, it must find out what works and what does not, and try to get faulty aspects to function more sensibly. Markets may be one way of doing this, but they are not a panacea. Much of what works and what does not has been known for a long time. While more research is necessary, it is not lack of knowledge *per se* that inhibits action, but a reluctance to act on existing knowledge.

Second, in order to achieve greater efficiency and control costs, it is absolutely crucial to manage the capacity of the system, because health care is fundamentally a capacity-driven system — if beds are built, people will fill them. It is also true that however many workers are trained, they will all find uses for their talents. There is, in general, no tendency for the system to get saturated. Technological innovation also seems to generate its own market, whether that be in new drugs or in high-tech equipment.

Capacity must be managed on three levels: physical, human and technological. There is already some measure of success on the first, and progress on the second, but Canada is currently failing with the third. Whatever management structures are created or modified, capacity must be adjusted to reflect desired outcomes. In the 1970s the nurse practitioner disappeared because of the over-supply of doctors. All of the available research said nurse practitioners were extremely effective and far cheaper than doctors. They did not survive because the other human capacities were not adjusted to make room for them.

This discussion of capacity is a caution that can be applied to any kind of reform. In an internal market context, the issue of capacity must be considered as a separate management burden. Like the pseudo-market of fee-for-service doctors and budgeted hospitals, the market itself does not limit capacity. It can, however, help promote efficiency when capacity is reduced, such as in the case of bed closures.

Third, management must achieve a firm consensus on the need for change. How can the consensus required for reform be reached? What is clear is that it cannot be achieved in a highly conflictual environment, because consensus requires getting information to providers and voters. It is currently apparent from the US experience that anyone who wants to stop reform does not have to prove that it is flawed, but simply has to generate enough confusion to keep the *status quo* from being changed. That confusion is easy to generate in a conflictual environment.

Whatever might be done with internal markets has to be embedded in a framework that allows bridges to be built from payers to providers. It cannot be all arm's length and heavy slugging, or the reforms will not succeed. Unless a sufficient level of understanding among providers and users can be achieved concerning why it is necessary to make changes, then the system will end up where it was in the 1960s; the potential benefit of reforms will be gone, and, given the current climate, the development of parasitic or parallel private markets will be more likely.

The Dangers of Doing Nothing

The danger of fully private markets is genuine and legitimate. The potential rewards of private entry into health care provision, where profits can be privatized and losses socialized, are enormous. Canada is unlikely to end up like the US, but the existing system could be eroded through failure to achieve a consensus. The implication is that there is probably little room for a major overhaul, but lots of potential for piecemeal, carefully targeted, and carefully thought-out changes in incentives.

The need for consensus is paramount, but the possibility of deterioration of the system during the potentially long consensus-building period is also important. This, again, suggests a need for progressive *ad hoc* modifications to the existing system rather than a complete refurbishing. To return to the German pharmaceutical example, the initial effort was to do something about costs, which worked. The pharmaceutical companies were dead set against the reforms, and for good reason; fewer prescriptions mean smaller profits. Industry people were presumably wringing their hands about how terrible it was to introduce effective policy when all of the necessary research on health outcomes had not yet been completed. Any action that is contingent on all the research first coming in will, of course, never occur.

The deeper message here is that consensus is crucial but unanimity is unlikely. Any effective policy to try to change patterns of utilization, and particularly to try to contain it, is going to hurt somebody. It is sensible to expect that whoever is hurt by changes will do their best to reverse the policy and to cause enough confusion to generate conflict. Successful reform will require not only an attempt to generate broad support, but the courage to implement sensible policies in the face of strong resistance from one quarter or another.

Åke Blomqvist was born in Sweden, where he pursued his undergraduate education at the Stockholm School of Economics. He received his Ph.D. in Economics from Princeton University. Since 1968, Dr. Blomqvist has taught at the University of Western Ontario, where he is currently a Professor in the Economics Department. His research has focussed on the economics of developing countries and the economics of health care. Dr. Blomqvist's work in health care economics has had an international flavour: his publications include an early monograph comparing health care policy in Canada, the United States and the United Kingdom; a number of papers in scientific journals; and an edited volume, published in 1994, on a range of issues in health care management in Canada and other countries.

Robert G. Evans is Professor of Economics and Senior Research Associate of the Centre for Health Services and Policy Research, University of British Columbia. He has been Commissioner of the British Columbia Royal Commission on Health Care and Costs (1990–91) and a member of the International Panel Review of the Swedish Health Care System (1991). He is a member of the Board of Editors of numerous health care journals and is currently Fellow and Director of the Canadian Institute for Advanced Research Program in Population Health. Professor Evans has been working in the field of health economics for more than 20 years and has published numerous books and articles on the subject.

Claude E. Forget is an independent consultant with a special interest in regulatory affairs, public policy analysis and business strategies in the financial and telecommunications sectors. After studying law in Canada and economics in both England and the United States, he taught economics at several Montreal universities. Mr. Forget has worked in the Quebec public sector in various policy-making roles, first as Assistant Deputy Minister and later as Minister and Member of the Legislative Assembly (1971–81). From 1983 to 1989 Mr. Forget was senior partner in the strategic planning and policy analysis consulting firm SECOR.

During that period, he chaired the Commission of Enquiry into the Canadian Unemployment Insurance Program. Most recently, he was Senior Vice President for corporate affairs of a financial group active in insurance and banking. During his career, Mr. Forget has been involved in several organizations, including the Civil Liberties Union (1966–68), the C. D. Howe Institute (1983–88), and the Asbestos Institute (1987–89). He is a member of the Quebec Medical Technologies Evaluation Board and is Chairman of the Royal Victoria Hospital, Montreal.

Howard Glennerster is Professor of Social Policy at the London School of Economics (LSE) and Chairman of the Suntory-Toyota International Centre for Economics and Related Disciplines at the LSE. He has worked on the finance of social welfare systems for many years and is author of *Paying for Welfare: The 1990s.* Professor Glennerster has just completed a study of the British NHS Reforms, supported by the King's Fund, looking especially at GP fundholding. His book *Implementing GP Fundholding* was published by Open University Press in October 1994.

Vivian Hamilton is a Medical Scientist at the Centre for the Analysis of Cost Effective Care and the Division of Clinical Epidemiology, Montreal General Hospital. She is also Assistant Professor in the departments of Medicine and Economics at McGill University. Her interests include cost-effectiveness analyses, utilization studies, regulatory health economics and studies of the effects of alcohol in the workplace. Dr. Hamilton has published several studies on the regulatory effects of the Medicare Hospice Benefit in the United States. She is currently conducting an analysis of the cost effectiveness of using computerized coronary risk profiles *versus* the Canadian Consensus Guidelines to identify and treat patients at high risk of hyperlipidaemia. Other projects include an assessment of the costs associated with waiting for coronary artery bypass graft surgery, comparisons of the utilization of health care services in Canada and the US and the effect of heavy drinking on earnings.

Monique Jérôme-Forget is President of the Institute for Research on Public Policy. She completed her Ph.D. in Psychology at McGill University in 1976. Since then, she has had a distinguished career in public service and in academia, having served as President of the Quebec

Workers' Compensation Board and Occupational Health and Safety Commission (Commission de la santé et de la sécurité au travail) and as an Assistant Deputy Minister at Health and Welfare Canada. During her academic career, Dr. Jérôme-Forget worked at McGill as an Adjunct Professor (1990–91) and at Concordia University, where she served as Vice-Rector in 1985–86. Dr. Jérôme-Forget is also an advisor to Statistics Canada.

Alan Maynard is Professor of Economics and Director of the Centre for Health Economics at the University of York. He has taught at the University of York since 1971 and has served in an advisory or consulting capacity for the World Health Organisation, the European Commission, the Organisation for Economic Co-operation and Development and the World Bank. He was a member of the British Economic and Social Research Council (ESRC) from 1986 to 1988 and of the Health Services Research Committee of the British Medical Research Council from 1986 to 1992. Professor Maynard was Chairman of the Evaluation Panel of the 4th Medical and Health Research Programme of the European Commission from 1989 to 1990. He was recently made a member of the ESRC Research Evaluation Steering Group. He is also a non-executive director of York NHS Hospital Trust and was for 10 years a member of York District Health Authority.

Clas Rehnberg is Assistant Professor at the Stockholm School of Economics. He received his Ph.D. in health economics from Linköping University in 1990, winning the 1991 Jan Blanpain Award for his thesis, "The Organization of Public Health Care: An Economic Analysis of the Swedish Health Care System." He has worked as a consultant for the Ministry of Finance and recently has been part of a group of experts analyzing options for changing the funding and organization of the Swedish health care system. Dr. Rehnberg has written articles on health care reform in Sweden as well as comparative analyses of the American, Canadian, and British systems. His current research interests include the application of institutional economics in the field of health care and health care policy.

Richard B. Saltman is Associate Professor and Director of the Division of Health Policy and Management at the Emory University

School of Public Health in Atlanta, Georgia. His research focusses on the behaviour of publicly operated health systems in Northern Europe, particularly in the Nordic region. He has been a consultant to health reform projects for the World Health Organisation, the Organisation for Economic Co-operation and Development and the World Bank. Most recently, he is co-editor, with Casten von Otter, of *Implementing Planned Markets in Health Care: Balancing Social and Economic Responsibilities,* which will be published by Open University Press in early 1995.

Frederik T. Schut is Assistant Professor of Health Economics in the Department of Health Policy and Management (BMG) at Erasmus University in Rotterdam. He teaches courses on health economics and on the structure, financing and organization of health care systems. He is involved in several research projects on health care reform, competition policy in health care and adverse selection in health insurance markets.

Wynand P. M. M. van de Ven is Professor of Health Insurance at Erasmus University in Rotterdam. His research activities are closely linked with the current reforms of the Dutch health care system. Professor van de Ven's major areas of research interest are: regulated competition in health care, competitive health insurance markets, adverse selection, moral hazard, cream skimming, risk-adjusted capitation payments, competition policy, managed care and econometrics. He has served on the Board of Directors of a hospital and a sickness fund and is a consultant to several health care organizations. As a visiting consultant, he has studied the health care systems of Sweden, Russia, Poland, Israel and New Zealand.

Joseph White is a Research Associate in the Governmental Studies programme at the Brookings Institution. His research interests include American budget policy and politics, Congress and entitlement programmes, especially health care. He is co-author, with Aaron Wildavsky, of *The Deficit and the Public Interest: The Search for Responsible Budgeting in the 1980s.* Dr. White's most recent book, *Competing Solutions: American Health Care Proposals and International Experience,* will be published by Brookings in 1995.

Joshua M. Wiener is a Senior Fellow in the Economic Studies programme at the Brookings Institution, where he specializes in health policy. During 1993, he worked for the White House Task Force on National Health Care Reform. Dr. Wiener has published five books and numerous articles on the organization, financing and delivery of long-term care, health care reform, rationing health care and improving access to health services for children and pregnant women. His latest book, *Sharing the Burden: Strategies for Public and Private Long-Term Care Insurance,* was published in May 1994.

SOCIAL POLICY

Ross Finnie, *Child Support: The Guideline Options*
Elisabeth B. Reynolds (ed.), *Income Security: Changing Needs, Changing Means*
Jean-Michel Cousineau, *La Pauvreté et l'État: Pour un nouveau partage des compétences en matière de sécurité sociale*
Choices/Choix — Social Security Reform:
    IRPP prend position / The IRPP Position
    Commentaries on the Axworthy Green Paper

OTHER IRPP PUBLICATIONS

City-Regions:
    Andrew Sancton, *Governing Canada's City-Regions: Adapting Form to Function*
    William Coffey, *The Evolution of Canada's Metropolitan Economies*
Education:
    Bruce Wilkinson, *Educational Choice: Necessary But Not Sufficient*
    Peter Coleman, *Learning About Schools: What Parents Need to Know and How They Can Find Out*
    Edwin G. West, *Ending the Squeeze on Universities*
Governance:
    Donald G. Lenihan, Gordon Robertson, Roger Tassé, *Canada: Reclaiming the Middle Ground*
    F. Leslie Seidle (ed.), *Seeking a New Canadian Partnership: Asymmetrical and Confederal Options*
    F. Leslie Seidle (ed.), *Equity and Community: The Charter, Interest Advocacy and Representation*
    F. Leslie Seidle (ed.), *Rethinking Government: Reform or Reinvention?*
Public Finance:
    Paul A.R. Hobson and France St-Hilaire, *Toward Sustainable Federalism: Reforming Federal-Provincial Fiscal Arrangements*

These and other IRPP publications are available from:
Renouf Publishing
1294 Algoma Road
Ottawa, Ontario
K1B 3W8
Tel.: (613) 741-4333   Fax.: (613) 741-5439